THE McCOLLOUGH EFFECT

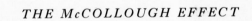

THE McCOLLOUGH EFFECT

An indicator of central neurotransmitter activity

C. C. D. SHUTE

Professor of Histology, Cambridge University
Fellow of Christ's College Cambridge

CAMBRIDGE UNIVERSITY PRESS

CAMBRIDGE

LONDON · NEW YORK · MELBOURNE

Published by the Syndics of the Cambridge University Press
The Pitt Building, Trumpington Street, Cambridge CB2 1RP
Bentley House, 200 Euston Road, London NW1 2DB
32 East 57th Street, New York, NY 10022, USA
296 Beaconsfield Parade, Middle Park, Melbourne 3206, Australia

First published 1979

Printed in Great Britain
at the University Press, Cambridge

Library of Congress cataloguing in publication data
Shute, Charles Cameron Donald, 1917–
The McCollough effect
Bibliography: p. 134   Includes index
1. Visual perception 2. Pattern perception 3. Neural transmission 4. Colour
vision
I. Title
QP492.S58   152.1′4   78–15609
ISBN 0 521 22395 4

CONTENTS

ACKNOWLEDGEMENTS

I wish to thank Dr Fergus Campbell, FRS, Dr Colin Blakemore, Professor John Ross, Professor Matt. Alpern, Professor Donald MacKay, Dr Keith White, Mr Larry Amure and Mr John Haldane for helpful discussions; my students for acting as subjects; Miss Fiona Hake for drawing the illustrations; Messrs Peter Joyce and Brian Secker for making the equipment; Miss Jane Allsup for doing the typing; and members of the staff of Cambridge University Press for seeing this book through publication.

This book is dedicated to
all those who love to observe, measure,
calculate and think

INTRODUCTION

Scope of the present work

This work is a study of one of the most extraordinary and mysterious of all visual phenomena – that known by the name of its discoverer Celeste McCollough. Many such psychophysical effects may be regarded as little more than laboratory curiosities, not necessarily of great importance in everyday life. The McCollough effect certainly involves 'phantom' colours, i.e. colours generated within the visual system of the brain rather than resulting from the character of the light reaching the eye, but nevertheless has properties that make one unwilling to accord it the status of a mere optical illusion. Of course, even illusions can form valuable objects of study, since the perceptual confusions resulting from particular external influences may reveal unsuspected aspects of the sensory processes themselves. Like illusions, the McCollough effect, although mainly passing unnoticed, may intrude itself on consciousness as an unsought and unwelcome part of one's visual experience. Mostly, however, to be aware of it one has to look for it. Its most significant feature – one not appreciated by its original discoverer – is the long period during which the effect can remain latent as a potential happening before it is actually evoked. It is as if the visual system has been, as it were, programmed to behave in this particular way, whereupon the capacity to do so is stored almost intact until the effective stimulus occurs to call forth the response. From this time on the power to respond declines, rapidly at first then more slowly, until after hours, days or weeks the effect can no longer be detected. Such a sequence of events strongly suggests an underlying purpose, the nature of which is perhaps easier to guess at than that of the underlying mechanisms involved.

The experiments about to be described have been mainly undertaken in an attempt to throw light on these mechanisms. The heavy emphasis on my own researches is not intended to belittle the work of others in the field. Not surprisingly, the subject has aroused enormous interest in many circles, and I cannot hope to do justice to all the observations that have been reported, particularly as these are not always consistent with one another. A main impediment to advance has been, I believe, the lack of a wholly satisfactory measuring method. To me, the phantom colours produced in the McCollough effect have seemed to possess features in common with interference colours, and for this reason I have in my method used for matching purposes the colours produced in birefringent material with polarised light. Unfortunately, interference colours are often neglected in texts on physical optics, and may be treated quite summarily even in works on crystallography where they are of particular importance. Because of this, I have considered the genesis of interference colours in some detail here, and have given a number of practical applications which, though not directly relevant to the main theme, may have some intrinsic interest in their own right and at the same time show how the suppression of certain wavelengths of light can produce, in varying circumstances, effects comparable to McCollough colours.

The McCollough effect, although mainly concerned with the way in which we perceive pattern and colour, has implications that are relevant to little-understood processes underlying memory, learning and forgetting. Because memory and learning are influenced by certain drugs, I have given particular attention to the influence exerted by these drugs on the McCollough effect, both on its initial strength and on its subsequent rate of decay. Does the McCollough effect also react to more normal factors, mirror perhaps the day-to-day or hour-to-hour variations in our psychic states of which we are all dimly aware? Are there characteristic responses to stress, patterns that can be associated with specific personality types, or changes induced by mental disease? If these and similar questions are to be answered, many measurements are required on many individuals. I have tried to begin such a study, and to provide a base-line with observations carried out on myself.

Aims and objects

My interest in the McCollough effect stems from work carried out over many years with my friend and colleague Dr Peter Lewis on the distribution of cholinergic pathways in the brain. Cholinergic pathways are those which produce their effects by releasing acetylcholine as a neurotransmitter from the nerve terminals. In student days I was inspired by the work of my teacher and supervisor Dr W. Feldberg on release of acetylcholine by nerve endings on muscle, and since that time I have hoped that cholinergic nerves might also be shown to occur wholly within the central nervous system. The first central cholinergic pathway to be discovered, through a technique which combined neurosurgery with neurohistochemistry (Shute and Lewis, 1961), was afferent to the hippocampus – a part of the brain which, in man at least, is essential to the laying down or retrieval of memories. The original histochemical method was directed at the not completely specific enzyme acetylcholinesterase, but later work (Lewis *et al.*, 1967) involving the more specific choline acetyltransferase confirmed the previous findings. Since then, many similar pathways have been revealed and mapped (Shute and Lewis, 1963, 1967; Lewis and Shute, 1967); some are shown in fig. 43(*a*). In the meantime Swedish workers (Dahlström and Fuxe, 1964; Fuxe, 1965) started to use a fluorescent technique, sometimes combined with surgery to uncover central pathways which use catecholamines (noradrenaline, dopamine) and the indoleamine 5-hydroxytryptamine as neurotransmitters. In this way a pattern began to emerge of so-called 'modulatory' systems controlling neural activity in many parts of the brain. As in the periphery, the noradrenaline system differs from the acetylcholine system in being highly divergent, and so must produce generalised rather than focal effects. Pharmacological studies have shown that in many regions acetylcholine has an excitatory effect on cell firing, whereas catecholamines and indoleamine are usually inhibitory. A number of inhibitory pathways and many inhibitory interneurones have since been found to use gamma-aminobutyric acid (GABA) as a neurotransmitter. Unfortunately, what neurotransmitters are released by terminals of the main, as opposed to modulatory, projection pathways of the brain (e.g. the sensory and motor tracts) is still uncertain. In some ways, however, the modulatory pathways are the more interesting and important, since they are less stable and respond more readily to external influences.

For a summary of the distribution and possible functions of the central pathways that make use of specific neurotransmitter substances, see Shute (1975) and Lewis and Shute (1978). Almost all brain regions come under the influence of the modulatory systems, including visual relays; nevertheless, it is not always easy to be sure of their effects in terms of behaviour. Although acetylcholine is predominantly excitatory and catecholamines (and 5-hydroxytryptamine) predominantly inhibitory at a cellular level, in behavioural terms their effects may be the opposite, through the intervention of an inhibitory relay. The dopamine system is depressed or destroyed in Parkinson's disease, and is thought to be at least relatively hyperactive in some psychotic states. The acetylcholine system is probably active in attention and arousal, learning and memory, and in dreaming sleep. There is, however, no means of showing in a direct way changing levels of modulatory activity in the living and behaving individual. Clearly it would be desirable if a measureable psychophysical phenomenon could be found to act as a marker of such activity. Could it be that the McCollough effect might fill this need?

These, then, have been my aims: to monitor cholinergic and other regulatory brain activity; to get a better understanding of the nature and function of the McCollough effect; to gain insights into perceptual and other higher mental processes generally. It is my hope that the simplicity of the apparatus, so cheap to construct and easy to transport, will encourage others, and not only professional physiologists and psychologists, to enter this fascinating field.

Addendum

Since the experiments described in this work are psychophysical in nature, they give little indication where in the visual system the postulated mechanisms may be occurring. Michael (1978, *J. Neurophysiol.* **41**, 1233–49) has recently described monocularly driven, colour sensitive, orientation selective simple cells in layer IV of the primate visual cortex. Although it is likely that cells such as these have an important function in relation to the McCollough effect, rather complex interactions with other neural systems are probably necessary to account for all its multifarious aspects.

1

THE McCOLLOUGH EFFECT

Original formulation

Celeste McCollough in her short but classic paper (McCollough, 1965) described how observers, having been presented with alternate projections of vertical and horizontal square-wave gratings on, respectively, an 'orange' and 'blue' background produced with coloured filters, on seeing a subsequent test pattern consisting of a vertical grating beside a horizontal one, reported an orange after-effect associated with the horizontal portion and a blue-green after-effect associated with the vertical portion of the pattern. The test pattern can be projected onto a screen, or may simply consist of white chalk lines on a blackboard, indicating what many workers have subsequently confirmed, that to evoke the phantom colours the test stimulus need not have a high luminance. When the test pattern consisted of curved or radiating lines rather than gratings, the colours were seen in association with the vertical and horizontal parts of the pattern only. The location of the colours was determined by the direction of the lines of the pattern; it did not change when the subject shifted his gaze so as to fixate on different regions. The colours did switch over, however, if either the pattern or the subject's head was turned through a right angle, and could be made to disappear with a rotation of 45°. The choice of adapting colours was not found to be crucial; distinguishable coloured after-effects could be obtained with almost any pair of filters that had different transmission characters. The after-effects were less saturated (i.e. more diluted with white) than typical negative after-images, but were longer lasting; that is to say, they persisted 'an hour or more' before totally disappearing.

McCollough carried out experiments to show that the coloured after-effects were set up independently by the two eyes without interocular transfer. Subjects adapted the left eye to an orange-vertical, blue-horizontal stimulus, tested each eye, then adapted the right eye to an orange-horizontal, blue-vertical stimulus and tested again. Most subjects as a result of this procedure saw reversed colours in the two eyes, i.e. orange associated with horizontal and green with vertical in the left, and orange associated with vertical and green with horizontal in the right. In most cases there was no interocular transfer from the adapted left eye to the unadapted right eye, but one subject did see, in the right eye before adaptation, the colours just obtained by adaptation of the left eye. In this instance, therefore, interocular transfer did occur.

McCollough also found that white light was not essential for the production of the coloured after-effects; they were still seen when the test pattern was viewed in nearly monochromatic green, yellow or orange light. I have partly confirmed this observation myself by setting up a McCollough effect in the manner described in chapter 3, and viewing the test pattern, consisting of a central grating orientated so as to evoke red surrounded by a peripheral grating orientated so as to evoke green, through a green filter which passed no red light. The central test area was seen as faintly reddened so long as the peripheral green area was kept in view to provide simultaneous colour contrast. When the periphery was masked this reddening was no longer detectable, and the central area reverted to green.

McCollough's remarkable observations were not entirely without precursors. She herself compared them to the complementary phantom fringes that replace the coloured fringes along the edges of objects produced by the wearing of prismatic spectacles (Kohler, 1962; Hay *et al.*, 1963). Meanwhile Hubel and Wiesel (1959, 1962) had showed that the visual cortex of cat contains cells that respond specifically to objects in the visual field presenting edges orientated in a particular direction. McCollough suggested that orientation-specific edge-detectors in the human visual system might be colour-coded, and subject to colour adaptation so that they come to respond with reduced sensitivity to those wavelengths with which they had previously been most strongly stimulated. On this hypothesis, only one class of receptive units is required to account for the McCollough effect.

Subsequent modifications and developments

Adapting colours

Some writers have preferred to drop the eponym, and refer to the McCollough effect as a particular type of contingent coloured after-effect, to be grouped with other subjective phenomena such as movement after-effects in which a given stimulus evokes a compensatory type of visual response. I shall continue with the eponymous usage, however, since it is widely known, and in later chapters, when units of strength are being applied to the red component, I shall employ the abbreviation ME.

Most authors state that they have used 'red' and 'green' adapting colours rather than the orange and blue of McCollough, but the difference in terms of the actual transmittance of their filters is less great than it sounds. The spectral transmission curve of McCollough's 'orange' Wratten filter does not peak in the orange region, but like most red filters other than interference filters forms a plateau, which in this instance occupies the red end of the spectrum as far back as the orange (610 nm). The colour transmitted is seen as red (it is so described by the manufacturers) or as orange-red if compared with a red filter which holds back wavelengths below, say 640 nm. McCollough's 'blue' filter peaks at 480 nm and gives a high transmission in the 460–500 nm range, i.e. it extends into the spectral turquoise region. The colour of this filter is described by the manufacturers as 'light blue-green'.

Many workers (e.g. Piggins and Leppman, 1973; Riggs *et al.*, 1974; Skowbo *et al.*, 1974; Uhlarik and Osgood, 1974; Jones and Holding, 1975) have preferred to pair a green filter with a magenta filter, on the grounds, presumably, that colour pairs would be more effective in eliciting the McCollough effect if they were complementary. The spectral sensitivities of the three types of retinal cone are such that when green light is viewed, the green receptors are activated in excess of the blue $(G > B)$, whereas when magenta (as opposed to purple) light is viewed, the red receptors are activated in excess of the blue $(R > B)$. Green and magenta in combination form white $(G > B + R > B = B + G + R = W)$; other complementary colour pairs can be designated in the same way (fig. 1 – colour pentagon 'A'). McCollough's paired colours can be regarded as approximately complementary, that is to say, in a chromaticity chart a line joining wavelengths of 480 nm and 610 nm passes through or close to the white point. She chose her particular filters

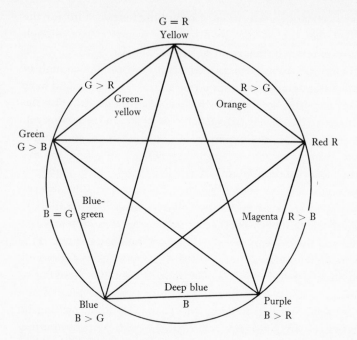

Fig. 1. Colour pentagon 'A'. Complementary colours, sited at apices and opposite sides. B, G, R indicate relative activation of blue, green and red retinal receptors.

to avoid an overlap of light in the yellow region. It is doubtful whether any particular advantage accrues from using magenta, and indeed the success of green–magenta combinations probably stems from the replacing of blue-green with green, rather than from substituting magenta for red. I have experimented with various filter combinations in an attempt to discover which are most efficacious in eliciting McCollough effects, i.e. which will produce the strongest effects in the shortest time. The best results were obtained, both in myself and in subjects who experience difficulty in seeing the McCollough effect, with the Wratten no. 25 orange-red filter as used by McCollough, combined with a Wratten no. 58 green filter (transmission peak at 530 nm). Although these colours are not complementary, the green coincides with the maximum spectral sensitivity of the green retinal receptors, and the orange-red is as close to the sensitivity peak of the red receptors (which is located in the yellow region of the spectrum) as it is possible to go while still retaining a sensation of red. This may account for the efficacy of the combination in producing a strong McCollough effect after a relatively short period of adaptation.

Subsequent workers have, in general, followed McCollough in projecting the coloured gratings alternately onto a screen, and have carefully controlled not only the total adaptation time, but also the time of exposure of each grating and the inter-grating time interval. I have not found, in my experiments, that this rigid procedure, which requires fairly elaborate apparatus, is necessary. A mains-operated slide-viewer, in which the coloured gratings are displayed side by side, is just as effective as a projection screen. The subject is asked to look at the gratings alternately for about 5 seconds each, as judged by counting from 'one hundred and one' to 'one hundred and five', for a total period of 5 minutes measured on a clockwork timer. It does not in the least matter if the observer is aware of one grating in his peripheral visual field while looking at the other, and he may fixate or not as he chooses. A McCollough effect can, in fact, be readily elicited in a naive audience sitting in a darkened or semi-darkened lecture threatre if paired coloured gratings are projected onto a screen with no instructions given whatsoever. Natural curiosity will cause most of those present to look at the screen, and that is enough.

Coloured gratings reproduced on the printed page are also adequate to set up a McCollough effect, if they are strongly illuminated (see Favreau and Cornwallis in *Scientific American*, December 1976). I have made effective gratings by sticking suitably aligned black-striped transparent adhesive tape over reflecting coloured foil. The achromatic test gratings do not need to be strongly lit, as has often been noted (Stromeyer, 1971; Skowbo *et al.*, 1974; White, 1976). Excessive illumination of the test pattern tends to suppress the McCollough effect, as does prolonged viewing of it. On the other hand, repeated rotation of the test pattern through 90° so as to alternate the induced colours is a useful method of intensifying them, particularly in subjects who only see faint McCollough effects. Probably the act of perceiving a particular McCollough colour fatigues that colour channel and sensitises the opponent channel, so that when the pattern is switched, the opposite McCollough colour is seen more strongly.

Adapting and test patterns

The gratings used to produce a McCollough effect need not be orientated vertically and horizontally. MacKay and MacKay (1974) habitually use left-oblique and right-oblique gratings, on the grounds, it appears, that these directional stimuli are less often encountered in everyday life. For most purposes, however, it does not matter if the subject already possesses a small McCollough effect before the onset of the experiment. As will be shown later (chapter 5), the behaviour of the McCollough effect set up as a result of the experimental procedure will be determined by the eventual strength achieved, irrespective of any bias in one direction or the other that may have been present before. Nor is it necessary for the adapting stimulus to consist of orthogonal straight-line gratings. Riggs (1973) found that curved lines in the same axis, convex upwards and concave upwards associated with red and green respectively, did almost as well, when tested with a pattern containing these two types of curvature, as rectilinear arrays with a directional contrast. Whether specific 'curvature detectors' need be postulated has been challenged (Stromeyer, 1974; Sigel and Nachmias, 1975), but McCollough effects can be obtained with pattern contrasts even more remote from that provided by gratings. MacKay and MacKay (1975a) found dot patterns with contrasting dot size effective, although the coloured after-effects were not as strong as those obtained with gratings. Even pattern and colour contrast in the adapting stimulus may not be necessary to produce a McCollough-like effect. A colleague has described to me how, after he had worked intensively with a calculator having a red illuminated digital display, many small colourless light-reflecting objects, and especially the white numbers registering competitors' times in a sporting programme shown on a black and white television set, appeared as an intense green. This seems to be an example of a spontaneous non-redundant McCollough effect (see chapter 5).

Another feature of gratings rather less potent than bar direction that can evoke a McCollough effect is spatial frequency. Lovegrove and Over (1972) found that uni-directional (vertical) gratings of different spatial frequency paired with red and green would evoke colour after-effects from similar achromatic test gratings, so long as the gratings differed in spatial frequency by an octave or more and the frequency of at least one grating exceeded 3 cycles per degree. Comparable results were obtained by Breitmeyer and Cooper (1972), while Leppman (1973) produced McCollough effects with concentric circles differing in spatial frequency. Various workers, e.g. Teft and Clark (1968), Stromeyer (1972a) have stated that McCollough effects produced by orthogonal gratings are spatial frequency specific, that is to say that strongest after-effects occur when the spatial frequency of the test grating matches that of the adopting gratings. Stromeyer found the most effective spatial frequency for eliciting the McCollough effect to be 5 cycles per degree. Uhlarik and Osgood (1974), however, varied bar widths and inter-bar spaces independently in the adaptation and test patterns and concluded that the most important determining factor was not spatial frequency but bar width. When the bar and space width in the adapting pattern were the same, the strongest after-effects were obtained when the bar width in the test pattern was doubled: i.e. there was no spatial frequency specificity. I have found, using rather low frequencies of $1\frac{1}{3}-2\frac{1}{3}$ cycles per degree, that increasing bar width in the test pattern tends to enhance the McCollough effect, whereas increasing inter-bar space width dilutes it. Decreasing spatial frequency by viewing at a closer distance diminishes the McCollough effect, but increasing spatial frequency by viewing from further off increases it. This could be due to the changes in the apparent inter-bar space width, in which case bar space width is more important in determining McCollough effect strength than bar width. Or it may be that increasing the spatial frequency of the test pattern increases the effective density of the directional stimulus, over-riding the frequency discrepancy which has a less powerful influence on the McCollough effect particularly at low frequencies. In practice, when measuring McCollough effect strength by the method described in chapter 3, care must be taken not to move the eyes back from the pattern during testing, because this will cause an increase in strength which, once produced, will not immediately revert to the true level when the head returns to its proper position.

If the test gratings are rotated away from the vertical–horizontal axes, a critical point is reached after about 25° when the McCollough effect can no longer be seen. The stronger the after-effect is initially, the greater the angle required to cause disappearance. Teft and Clark (1968) exploited this property to provide a simple, if not too precise method of estimating relative McCollough effect strengths. I have found that increases in the strength of the McCollough effect can be detected with some sensitivity by using a test pattern with wider inter-bar spaces than those of the adapting pattern. The adapting gratings consisted of bars and spaces of equal width and when projected onto a screen at a distance of 2 metres gave a spatial frequency of 2 cycles per degree. In the test pattern the distance between the bars was twice the bar width, so that the spatial frequency was then $1\frac{1}{3}$ cycles per degree. Four subjects were tested; all had previously seen a distinct McCollough effect when tested with a 2 cycles per degree pattern matching the adapting pattern. With the $1\frac{1}{3}$ cycles per degree test pattern substituted, no coloured after-effect was seen until the subject retreated from the screen to reduce the effective spatial frequency and inter-bar width. If the subject then returned to the 2 metres position while still viewing the test grating, the McCollough effect was retained. It appears that once the after-effect has been perceived, a weaker stimulus will suffice to evoke it. The McCollough effect was allowed to decay, and the procedure was repeated $\frac{3}{4}$ hour after taking a drug (hyoscine: see chapter 7) which, in other subjects, had been found to enhance the McCollough effect. In all four cases the $1\frac{1}{3}$ cycles per degree test pattern now provoked a coloured after-effect which appeared subjectively to be as strong as that previously produced by the 2 cycles per degree pattern.

The phantom colours
In order that the induced colours should be seen most clearly, later workers have improved on McCollough's arrangement of two large orthogonal gratings side by side for the test pattern by devising arrays of multiple orthogonal gratings forming a kind of chequerboard. Since I have been concerned mainly in measuring one component of the McCollough effect, the red, in order to get maximum colour contrast I have adopted a test pattern consisting of a single triangular-shaped grating totally surrounded by an orthogonal grating. Brightness contrast is also important in eliciting the McCollough effect. It has been claimed that the after-effect remains strong even when the edges of the black bars in the test pattern are blurred by defocussing (Gibson and Harris, quoted by

.Murch, 1969), so that the phenomenon must be due to contrast rather than contours. This, however, is not true; careful measurement shows that the McCollough effect, though still present, is considerably weakened when the bar edges in the test pattern are not sharp. For this reason, it is necessary to ensure that subjects taking part in experiments not only possess normal colour vision but also do not have uncorrected refractive errors. Particular care must be taken with female subjects who, as is well known, are more likely to have uncorrected visual defects than men. Lightness and brightness contrast may affect the quality of the colours seen, as well as their intensity. Stromeyer (1971) used a chequer-board test pattern in which the grating units had bars that were various shades of grey rather than black, and spaces with similar shades instead of white, in random combinations. High contrast gratings, i.e. those with black bars and white spaces, gave rise to the usual red and green after-effects; but light gratings, i.e. those with grey bars, produced orange and yellow colours rather than red, and dark gratings, i.e. those with grey spaces, produced blue and violet colours rather than green. Stromeyer compared these 'distorted' McCollough colours with the colours that can be produced with two-colour projections (see Land, 1977).

Normal McCollough colours, i.e. those produced under standard conditions of light–dark contrast, are only approximately complementary to the adapting colours. Stromeyer (1969) surprisingly claimed that, whatever the adapting colours, the phantom colours evoked by them were always red and green. This view, which is certainly incorrect, he later retracted (Stromeyer, 1972a), although still maintaining that blues, yellows and oranges were 'not as readily produced'. In fact, good yellow and orange after-effects are obtained after adapting respectively to Wratten filters 47B (deep blue, peak transmittance 430 nm) and 45 (light blue, peak transmittance 480 nm). A blue after-effect is obtained with a Wratten orange filter 21, but since this transmits beyond 600 nm far into the red, better results can be obtained with an orange interference filter. I have measured the strengths of blue and orange McCollough effects in myself by the match interference method ($1\frac{1}{2}\lambda$ wave plates rotated between parallel polars, see chapter 3) and have found them to be as great as that of a red McCollough effect obtained with a similarly long adaptation period. This indicates that, although some subjects find red McCollough effects easiest to see, possibly because of the well-known attention-catching properties of red, nevertheless all colours linked to patterns are equipped to produce after-effects, and not preferentially green and red.

It is not essential for the adapting colours to be highly saturated in order to induce a McCollough effect: quite strong effects can be obtained with unsaturated colours, as one would expect if the mechanism operates in ordinary life, where most of the colours one sees are relatively unsaturated. Unless glass filters are specially obtained, coloured gratings projected onto a large screen for mass audiences require to be on photographic film, since gelatine filters are liable to melt. For this reason a high degree of saturation is impossible, yet good McCollough effects are obtained, particularly if the ambient illumination is low. For quantitative work, and for determining the actual McCollough hues, filters with a narrow transmission band are desirable. Apart from the Wratten filters already mentioned, I have used numbers 64 (blue-green, peak transmission 510 nm), 61 (green, peak transmission 525 nm), 29 (red, transmission 640 + nm) and 70 (far red, transmission 700 nm) and for a good source of yellow and deep blue-violet light I have employed a whole wave plate for yellow light, $\lambda = 580$ nm, between parallel and crossed polars respectively (see chapter 2). By combining the adapting colours in various ways (it is often easier to distinguish McCollough hues if they are not nearly complementary but relatively close to one another in Newton's scale), it was possible to draw up a table relating adapting colours to McCollough colours and to compare the latter with the complementaries of the adapting colours (table 1).

It will be seen from table 1 that the McCollough colour (McCollough 'complementary') is in general yellower than the true complementary of the adapting colour. This is also characteristic of the 'complementary' colour pairs that are seen when birefringent transparent material thick enough to cause interference is viewed between crossed and parallel polars. The birefringent 'complementaries' are in fact the same as the McCollough 'complementaries' (fig. 2 – colour pentagon 'B'). This correspondence gave me the idea that McCollough colours could have features in common with interference colours and might be measured by matching with them. Birefringence interference colours can be

Table 1

Adapting colour	McCollough colour	Complementary
Violet	Yellow	Green-yellow
Blue	Deep yellow	Orange
Blue-green	Orange	Red
Green	Red	Magenta
Deep yellow	Blue	Deep blue
Orange	Blue-green	Blue
Red	Green	Blue-green
Deep red	Green-yellow	Deep green

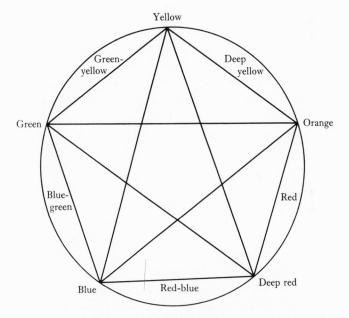

Fig. 2. Colour pentagon 'B'. Birefringence interference colours produced with crossed and parallel polars, sited at apices and opposite sides.

formed either as a result of extinction of certain wavelengths so that the spectral transmittance curve shows a minimum (destructive interference), or as a result of maximal transmission of a particular wavelength with progressively less transmission of adjacent wavelengths (constructive interference). If the birefringent material has its 'slow direction' (see chapter 2) at 45° to the transmission axes of the polars, the interference colours are too highly saturated to match with McCollough colours; but when the birefringent material is rotated away from the diagonal position so that the slow direction approaches the transmission axes of the polars, the interference colour becomes progressively desaturated. If a suitable thickness of birefringent material is chosen to give an appropriate 'retardation' and is rotated between parallel polars, all the McCollough colours listed in table 1 can be closely matched. This suggests that the colour corresponding to the wavelength whose destruction gives rise to a birefringent interference colour can be regarded as analogous to the adapting colour that generates the McCollough effect. In other words, the adapting colour sets up an inhibitory mechanism in the visual system whereby that colour is subsequently preferentially suppressed. But not all interference colours can be produced by destructive interference: interference green is due to constructive interference, i.e. maximal transmission of the corresponding wavelength. Since green McCollough effects are seen, it follows that another mechanism such as colour opponency must also be at work.

Storage

The more that is discovered about the McCollough effect, the harder it becomes to accept the original supposition that the after-effect is due to simple adaptation of single pattern- and colour-coded units in the visual system. Murch (1972) noted that an orientation-specific size after-effect, induced simultaneously with the McCollough orientation-specific colour after-effect, showed interocular transfer whereas the McCollough effect did not. He pointed out that colour-coded cells are located predominantly in the lateral geniculate body (Wiesel and Hubel, 1966) and orientation-specific edge-detectors predominantly in the visual cortex (Hubel and Wiesel, 1968) and suggested that an adaptation response occurring in the colour-sensitive geniculate cells was somehow 'fed into' the orientation-sensitive cortical cells. Skowbo *et al.* (1975) in a review article argued that the extraordinarily long persistence of the McCollough effect was against adaptation in the sense of fatigue of colour mechanisms being directly responsible for the phantom colours seen, and supported the view that McCollough effects should be regarded as learned responses. Murch (1976) put forward the view that the induction of a McCollough effect might be likened to classical conditioning. If a comparison is made with the Pavlovian situation whereby a dog responds to the unconditioned stimulus of food in the mouth by salivating (unconditioned response) and after conditioning with the sound of a bell makes the same (conditioned) response without the presence of the unconditioned stimulus, then in the McCollough analogue the unconditioned stimulus is the adapting colour, the unconditioned response is the negative after-image produced by that colour, the conditioned stimulus is the adapting and test pattern, and the conditioned response is the phantom colour reproducing the appearance of the negative after-image. Some pros and cons of the conditioning model are discussed by McCarter and Silver (1977) and Murch (1977); see also Mayhew and Anstis (1972).

One respect in which the McCollough effect does not wholly resemble conditioning relates to its decay. In conditioning, decay results from lack of presentation of the conditioning factors, i.e. to use the language of psychology, from lack of reinforcement. After decay has occurred, relatively few applications of the conditioning factors are required to restore the conditional state. Repeated presentation of the conditioned stimulus without the unconditioned stimulus leads to the extinction of the conditioning. Does the McCollough effect exhibit these three features of conditioning: decay, reinforcement and extinction? Jones and Holding (1975) and Holding and Jones (1976) have claimed that the McCollough effect does not undergo a significant amount of decay until it is first tested; that is to say, once the capacity to produce the after-effect is set up, that capacity is stored without further presentations of the adapting stimuli until it is called into play. Although Jones and Holding may have somewhat exaggerated the degree of storage, there is no doubt that the decay during the period between adaptation and first test, even though this be quite prolonged, is relatively much less than the loss of strength that occurs after the first test. MacKay and MacKay (1975*b*, 1977) found that loss of strength is arrested by darkness and sleep. Measuring the strengths of the individual McCollough colours, I was able to show that the red component of the after-effect is protected from degradation if red light is excluded from the eye, either with a green filter or with anti-laser interference glasses (Shute, 1977c). The green component can be similarly protected with a red filter, which will also cause the red component to lose strength more rapidly than normal (see chapters 3 and 4).

The waning of the McCollough effect after the first test is not strictly comparable with the extinction of conditioning, since the loss of strength does not merely ensue from the re-presentation of the adapting pattern, but from the pattern accompanied by colours that are opponent with respect to the adapting colours. If the seeing of these colours contributes to their eventual disappearance one might expect that they would disappear more rapidly the more frequent the testing. In the extreme cases, this appears to be true: if a subject has been tested only once, the after-effect may last for weeks, whereas if he gazes at the test pattern without intermission the phantom colours may be gone in 10–15 minutes. If the subject rotates his head or the test slide repeatedly through 90° so as to transpose the colours, they are enhanced and loss of strength is retarded. With regular testing every twelve minutes for 2–3 hours, I have usually found that the after-effect has disappeared or is very weak by next day. Increasing the test interval by three times did not significantly affect the rate of loss.

Almost all workers who habitually induce in themselves McCollough effects find that increasingly short adaptation times are required to do so. This may be compared with the 'reinforcement' of conditioning. It seems clear, however, that whatever likenesses may exist between conditioning and the McCollough effect, the latter has many features peculiar to itself that need to be studied in their own right, and no advantage is gained by trying to force them into a predetermined conceptual mould. For this reason I shall avoid the terminology of conditioning in describing the McCollough effect. I shall apply the term 'decay' to loss of strength occurring or presumed to occur at any stage after the initial exposure to colour and pattern, which I shall continue to call 'adaptation' in deference to time-honoured practice, although the usage may be regarded as not wholly appropriate and so liable to mislead.

2

INTERFERENCE COLOURS AND BIREFRINGENCE

Naming the colours

Since it is crucial to the argument of this book that the phantom colours of the McCollough effect have something in common with interference colours, and since interference colours are used to measure them, some consideration will be given in this chapter to the different ways in which interference colours can be formed. Those caused by destructive interference have a rather characteristic appearance on account of the unusual combination of wavelengths involved. Nevertheless there is no accepted nomenclature for distinguishing the various gradations of colour, other than the names applied to spectral colours. Text-book reproductions of the visible spectrum are notoriously unreliable. For instance (and I am indebted to Dr F. W. Campbell for drawing my attention to this curious fact) almost all of them show a wide band of yellow, and yet in a continuous spectrum no pure yellow can be seen: green-yellow merges imperceptibly into orange-yellow unless the yellow region around $\lambda = 572.5$ nm is isolated by masking. It is possible that the explanation is to be found in colour opponency mechanisms (see De Valois et al., 1966). In a discontinuous spectrum yellow is seen in the $\lambda = 572.5$ nm region as a result of approximately equal activation of green and red receptors ($G = R$). In the continuous spectrum, stimulation of the green receptors by the green region may inhibit the red receptors responding to the adjacent yellow region, converting $G = R$ to $G > R$ (green-yellow). Similarly, stimulation of the red receptors by the orange region may inhibit the green receptors responding to the yellow region adjacent to it,

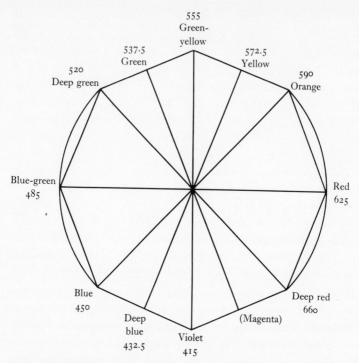

Fig. 3. Circular spectrum (colour octagon). Spectral wavelengths corresponding to violet, blue, blue-green, deep green, green-yellow, orange, red and deep red, separated by 35 nm. Complementary wavelengths separated by 140 nm.

converting G = R to R > G (orange-yellow). A temporary appearance of yellow in the green-yellow or orange-yellow region of the continuous spectrum can be produced by previously fatiguing the eye with green or red light respectively. Turquoise (due to B = G) is seen in the continuous spectrum because there is not a mutual antagonism or opponency between the blue and green mechanisms.

A useful guide to the location of spectral colours in the visible range of wavelengths from 400 nm to 700 nm is provided by the *Scientific American* version of the spectrum (Feinberg, 1968). This tour-de-force of printing is not completely faithful to the continuous spectrum as it is actually seen – for instance a distinct narrow band of yellow is shown – but it does site accurately the key positions of blue-green (turquoise), yellow and orange lights at $\lambda = 485$ nm,

$\lambda = 572.5$ nm and $\lambda = 590$ nm respectively. From this information it is possible to construct a circular or octagonal version of the spectrum with complementary colours at opposite points as shown in fig. 3. In this diagram, spectral wavelengths corresponding to violet, blue, blue-green, deep green, green-yellow, orange, red and deep red are separated by intervals of 35 nm, and complementary wavelengths by intervals of 140 nm. Magenta is included (in brackets) as the complementary of green although it is not a spectral colour. The wavelengths assigned to the blues and reds may be regarded as somewhat arbitrary since there is little colour contrast at the two ends of the spectrum, but the regular spacing is helpful in the analysis of interference colours.

The interference series of colours known as Newton's scale reflects the spectral series with reasonable closeness so that similar names can be used. The interference series, however, shows a distinct band of yellow: one of the reasons for regarding the rainbow as due in part to interference and not a pure spectrum is that yellow can be seen in it. Difficulties arise in the red region of the interference series. Spectral reds at the long wavelength end do not of course contain blue: they simply darken. The deepest interference red, on the other hand, has a considerable blue component, and could appropriately be called 'rose-red' or 'blush red'. Nevertheless, since such terms are not in general use, I shall avoid them. It is characteristic of the interference series that there is a sudden transition from deepest red to deepest blue. The region where this occurs is often known as the 'sensitive tint'.

Thin film interference colours

The best known interference colours are those produced by reflection of white light from the two surfaces of a thin film such as that made by oil spread on water or by soap bubbles. Interference colours are also formed by a thin film of air between two surfaces of glass, and as such were studied by Newton (*Opticks*, Book 2). To see interference colours made by a thin film of air, the reader need only take two clean glass slides as used for light microscopy, press them firmly together and view them by reflected light. He will see coloured rings due to light internally reflected off the back surface of the film interfering with light reflected from its front surface. Increasing the pressure causes the film to become thinner;

any pair of rings will move outwards, become more widely spaced, and new rings will appear within them. When the slides are tilted so as to increase the angle of incidence of the light, the path difference between the two reflected beams decreases and a shorter wavelength of light is reflected. With normal incidence the path difference is twice the optical thickness of the film (actual thickness multiplied by refractive index) and since the film is of air with a refractive index of unity, is equal to twice the actual thickness. There is a further complication that when light passes through a medium of lower refractive index to be reflected at an interface with a medium of higher refractive index, it is slowed by half a wavelength. As a result, constructive interference giving maximum reflectance of a particular wavelength λ occurs when twice the thickness of the film is equal to $\frac{1}{2}\lambda$, $\frac{3}{2}\lambda$, $\frac{5}{2}\lambda$ etc., i.e. when the thickness is $\frac{1}{4}\lambda$, $\frac{3}{4}\lambda$, $\frac{5}{4}\lambda$ etc. Destructive interference giving minimum reflectance, that is to say extinction, occurs when twice the thickness is λ, 2λ, 3λ etc., i.e. when the thickness is $\frac{1}{2}\lambda$, $\frac{3}{2}\lambda$ etc. In the case of a reflecting interference filter consisting of two silvered semi-reflecting glass plates separated by a spacer, the optical thickness of the spaces is made to be $\frac{1}{4}\lambda$ to reflect light of wavelength λ. With a transmission interference filter there is no phase change due to reflection, so that light of wavelength λ is maximally passed when the spacer has an optical thickness of $\frac{1}{2}\lambda$. If the filter is tilted through an angle θ, the wavelength maximally transmitted will be shortened to $\lambda \cos \theta$.

The optical system used by Newton for studying interference colours consisted of a convex lens with a long radius of curvature applied to a flat glass plate. The layer of air trapped between the two caused a series of coloured fringes now known as Newton's rings, with a central black spot when viewed by reflected light and a white spot with transmitted light. Newton gave the succession of colours in the innermost rings from within outwards as violet (purple), blue, green, yellow, red. With reflected light, he described a blue ring immediately outside the black spot, then white, yellow, red. Newton made similar observations on the colours reflected from soap bubbles and these he divided into Orders as follows: 1st Order, black, blue, white, yellow, orange, red; 2nd Order, violet, blue, green, yellow, orange, red, etc. He also included various shades of red and inserted 'indigo' between violet and blue so as to produce eight colours in each Order to match the musical notes of an octave: hence the term Newton's scale.

With knowledge of the wave theory of light it is possible to go beyond Newton and account for various features of his rings. The black spot at the centre of the reflected rings is due to the phase difference of $\frac{1}{2}\lambda$ imposed by the air–glass interface on all values of λ, causing destructive interference with the light reflected by the glass–air interface. The so-called 1st Order blue immediately surrounding the black spot is not in series with the other coloured rings. It is formed because the black spot is larger for lights of long wavelength than for lights of short wavelength, so that there is a relative suppression of orange and red light at the edge of the black spot, giving rise to the sensation of blue. Light of wavelength λ is minimally reflected at thicknesses of $\frac{1}{2}\lambda$, λ, $\frac{3}{2}\lambda$ etc. and maximally reflected at thicknesses of $\frac{1}{4}\lambda$, $\frac{3}{4}\lambda$, $\frac{5}{4}\lambda$ etc. Short wavelength light is the first to be maximally reflected, e.g. blue light $\lambda = 450$ nm at a thickness of $\frac{1}{4} \times 450 = 110$ nm, which accounts for the silvery white appearance outside the first blue ring. The yellow, orange and red of the 1st Order are due to minima for blue, blue-green and green light occurring at thicknesses of $\frac{1}{2} \times 450 = 225$ nm, $\frac{1}{2} \times 485 = 242.5$ nm, $\frac{1}{2} \times 537.5 = 270$ nm respectively. Newton's 2nd Order blue is due to minimum reflection of deep yellow and occurs at a thickness of $\frac{1}{2} \times 580 = 290$ nm. Since it is the first interference blue to be formed, it would be more appropriate to call it 1st Order blue, and have the series of interference colours run not from blue to red but from yellow to green.

Newton calculated and recorded the radius of curvature of his convex lens (91 inches) and measured the diameter of the fifth 'dark' ring (i.e. red–blue junction: 16/79 inches). The dark ring or red–blue junction is due to the suppression of yellow light. Since the radius of curvature R is large compared with the wavelength of yellow light, it follows from the geometry of the system that the diameter of the nth dark ring d_n is given by $d_n = 2\sqrt{(Rn\lambda)}$. Substituting the metric equivalents of Newton's values for R and d_5, we get $\lambda = 572.5$ nm, which is precisely the value that we have taken to be the wavelength of yellow light. Furthermore, the thickness t of film producing an nth Order dark ring due to extinction of light of wavelength λ is given by $t = \frac{1}{2}n\lambda$. Substituting $n = 5$, $\lambda = 572.5$ nm, we get $t = 1431.25$ nm. Newton calculated the thickness of the film at the 5th dark ring to be 32/567931 inches, which is 1431.2 nm. It is one of the great ironies of science that Newton had to hand measurements that could have established for him the wave theory of light.

One application of thin film interference enables one to judge the thickness of sections cut for electron microscopy as they float on the collecting trough. The optical thickness of a red section, whose colour is due to the extinction of green light $= \frac{1}{2} \times 537.5 = 270$ nm. Since the refractive index of the embedding material contained in the section $= 1.54$, the actual thickness $= 270/1.54 = 175$ nm. Similarly the optical thickness of a purple section (due to extinction of yellow light) $= \frac{1}{2} \times 572.5 = 285$ nm, so that the actual thickness $= 185$ nm. The optical thickness of a blue section (due to extinction of deep yellow) $= \frac{1}{2} \times 580 = 290$ nm, so that the actual thickness $= 190$ nm. The ideal section for electron microscopy is silver and has an actual thickness of 75 nm; the wavelength *maximally* reflected is $4 \times 1.54 \times 75 = 460$ nm (light blue).

Opals and cat's eyes

A multilayer reflecting interference filter consists of a series of thin films such that the optical thickness of each film and of the spaces between films is $\frac{1}{4}\lambda$. In this way the reflectivity of the system is greatly increased as compared with a single film. Nearly monochromatic reflection may also occur when the reflecting elements are not layers but spherical or even cylindrical bodies: light is then reflected off the front and back surfaces of the bodies to produce the interference. The loss of intensity due to the lack of continuous layers can be partly compensated for by increasing the number of reflecting elements. In such a system the wavelength of reflected light need not change, as it does when the reflecting elements are layered, with changes in the angle of incidence of the light.

Opal has been shown to consist of regularly stacked spherical particles of amorphous silica (Darragh *et al.*, 1976). These authors have suggested that the colours characteristic of precious opal result from the diffraction of light by the areas between the spheres according to Bragg's law for the scattering of X-rays by a crystal lattice. There appears to be little evidence that the inter-sphere spaces would diffract light in this way, or if they did so that they would produce the strong reflected spectral colours of opal.

Moreover, such a theory fails to take account of the $\frac{1}{2}\lambda$ phase change that occurs when light is reflected at a low to high refractive index interface. It seems much likelier that the colours of opal are due, not to the spaces, but to the spheres themselves reflecting from their front and back surfaces. Light from the front surface undergoes a $\frac{1}{2}\lambda$ phase change and constructively interferes with light retarded by $\frac{1}{2}$ or $\frac{3}{2}$ wavelengths. For normally incident light, these conditions are fulfilled when the optical thickness of the spheres is equal to $\frac{1}{4}$ or $\frac{3}{4}$ wavelengths. Maximal reflection of light in the visible range by spheres with the dimensions of those found in opal occurs when $\lambda = \frac{4}{3} \times$ optical thickness. Taking the refractive index of the amorphous silica to be 1.45, a deep blue ($\lambda = 425$ nm) will be produced by a sphere diameter of 220 nm, and a deep red ($\lambda = 675$ nm) by a sphere diameter of 350 nm. These figures fit well with the estimate by Darragh *et al.* of a sphere diameter range of 150–350 nm.

In the vertebrate eye, the reflecting layer behind the retina that is responsible for causing 'eye-shine' is called the tapetum lucidum. In fish and reptiles the reflecting elements of the tapetum are commonly crystals of guanine, and these have been shown to possess the dimensions, spacing and refractive index required to give multilayer interference (Land, 1966). A tapetum is present in mammals other than primates, and can be regarded as a relic of their evolutionary origin from nocturnal or crepuscular ancestors. In ungulates the tapetum is formed by collagen bundles, while in carnivores the reflecting elements consist of minute rodlets located in the cytoplasm of specialised tapetal cells. These rodlets appear to be arranged in an orderly way, but unlike the spheres of opal are not in close contact with one another, but instead are completely surrounded by cytoplasmic spaces. This shows that close-packing of the repeating elements is not required to produce a physical colour. Pedler (1963) argued unconvincingly that light was diffracted from a lattice formed by the centres of the rodlets. However, his estimate of their diameter was more than twice that reached by other workers before and since, his value for the refractive index was extremely low in view of the electron density of the rodlets, and the reflectivity peak of 600 nm that he ended up with, well into the orange, scarcely accords with the greenish-yellow colour typically seen in the cat tapetum. If, on the other hand, the rodlets have an average diameter of nearly 100 nm and their refractive index is about 1.4 as would result from a protein concentration approaching 50 per cent, their optical thickness would be 140 nm, and the light produced by constructive interference between the rays reflected from their front and back surfaces would have a wavelength of 560 nm, i.e. that of green-yellow.

Glories, coloured suns, blood-films

Certain rare but interesting meteorological phenomena can be explained in terms of interference. An anti-corona or 'glory' is sometimes seen around the shadow of an aeroplane cast on a cloud: an excellent coloured photograph with the dimensions of the halos recorded has been reproduced in *Scientific American* (Bryant and Jarmie, 1974). I have argued elsewhere (Shute, 1977a) that the coloured rings are due to light reflected back from the front and back surfaces of the deeper droplets of the cloud (these are too large to produce thin film interference) being diffracted by the more superficial droplets to form a so-called Airy diffraction pattern. The size of these droplets can be calculated. Measured in μm, their diameter is approximately equal to the cosecant of the angular radius of the innermost red ring of the Airy pattern, and in the case of Bryant and Jarmie's glory must have been close to 20 μm.

Coloured suns and moons, including the fabulous 'blue moon', may be due to an unusual type of interference first described by Thomas Young (1802) and known as 'mixed plate' interference, in which light traversing very small refractile elements interferes with light passing between them (Shute, 1976). If this is so, the water droplets responsible for a blue sun or moon will have a diameter of about 1 μm – these are about the smallest that occur in clouds. The phenomenon can also be caused by oil droplets produced by forest fires; because of their higher refractive index, the effective diameter is then only 0.7 μm.

Glory-like halos and a coloration due to mixed plate interference are both seen when a point source of white light is viewed through a blood smear held close to the eye. The halos result from diffraction of light by the flattened red cells, and the mean diameter of these cells can be calculated from the diameter of the rings (Campbell *et al.*, 1975). The light source in the centre of the halos is seen as coloured because the optical thickness of the red cells differs from that of the surrounding plasma. In an ideal blood film only one cell thick the colour is red, due to the extinction of green light ($\lambda = 535$ nm). If the film is tilted through $25°$, its effective thickness and therefore the wavelength extinguished is increased by sec $25°$ to become 590 nm, i.e. that of orange light. In consequence the colour changes to blue.

Birefringence

The most important type of interference in relation to the present study is that due to birefringence, and is produced with polarised light. The polarising microscope reveals interference colours when a transparent birefringent object of sufficient thickness is orientated in the 'diagonal position', that is to say, with its optical axis (a plane at right angles to this axis has the same refractive index in all directions) at $45°$ to the axis of transmission of the polariser and is viewed with the analyser in the crossed or parallel position. If the sign of the birefringence is positive, the optical axis is the 'slow direction', i.e. the direction of higher refractive index. The linearly polarised incident beam as it travels through the object is split into two component rays vibrating one in the plane of the optical axis (slow direction) and one at right angles to it. A phase difference is set up between the two rays because of the different optical densities in the two directions, so that when they leave the object, one is retarded with respect to the other. On account of this retardation, the emergent beam formed by the recombination of the fast and slow rays is elliptically polarised. For any given retardation, the component wavelengths of white light will emerge with different degrees of ellipticity, and so will be differentially held back by the analyser. The mixture of transmitted wavelengths will result in an interference colour characteristic of the retardation.

The relationship between retardation and the interference colours produced can be determined with a graduated quartz wedge (quartz is birefringent). Such a wedge has to be calibrated. This can be done by setting the wedge in the diagonal position between crossed or parallel polars and noting the distance between the extinction lines produced with a monochromatic green light source ($\lambda = 546$ nm) provided by a narrow-band Zeiss interference filter. In the wedge that I use, these extinction lines are 19 gradations apart on the graduated scale. This indicates that a single gradation represents a difference in retardation of $546 \div 19 = 29$ nm. Since light of wavelength λ is minimally transmitted at retardations of $n\lambda$ with crossed polars and at retardations of $\frac{1}{2}(2n+1)\lambda$ with parallel polars, n being integral, the position of each extinction line gives a measure of the retardation of the wedge at that point.

The calibrated quartz wedge can now be observed in the diagonal position between crossed and parallel polars with a white light source to show the sequence of interference colours. The transitions from red to blue, which are sharply demarcated, occur at a constant distance apart along the wedge equal to 20 gradations on the scale, representing a difference in retardation of $20/19 \times 546 = 575$ nm. The first red–blue junction seen with crossed polars occurs one gradation beyond the position of the first extinction line produced with green light, i.e. at a retardation of $546 + 29 = 575$ nm. This retardation is close enough to the value for the wavelength of yellow light ($\lambda = 572.5$) obtained from Newton's measurements. We can conclude that the red–blue junctional region in the interference sequence is generated when yellow light is minimally transmitted, at retardations equal to $n\lambda$ with crossed polars and $\frac{1}{2}(2n+1)\lambda$ with parallel polars, where λ is the wavelength of yellow light. Similarly, the interference colour light yellow occurs when yellow light is maximally transmitted, at retardations of $\frac{1}{2}(2n+1)\lambda$ with crossed polars and $n\lambda$ with parallel polars. This is in accordance with the rule that for any retardation, light minimally transmitted with crossed polars is maximally transmitted with parallel polars, and vice versa.

The relationship between other interference colours and the wavelengths of lights maximally and minimally transmitted can be determined in a similar manner. In fig. 3 the visible spectrum is subdivided into colours at 35 nm wavelength intervals as follows: violet (far blue) 415 nm; blue 450 nm; blue-green 485 nm; deep green 520 nm; green-yellow 555 nm; orange 590 nm; red 625 nm; deep red 660 nm. Retardations giving maximum and minimum transmission of these wavelengths ($R = n\lambda$ or $\frac{1}{2}(2n+1)\lambda$) are readily calculated, and the interference colours produced by their retardation with crossed and parallel polars can be observed on the quartz wedge. The results of this exercise are given in table 2, with retardations expressed to the nearest 5 nm. The table shows for each retardation the interference colour seen with crossed and parallel polars, and the wavelengths maximally and minimally

Table 2 *Retardations giving birefringence interference colours, ranging from 1st Order red–blue with parallel polars to 2nd Order red–blue with crossed polars*

Retardation (to nearest 5 nm)	Interference colour crossed polars	Min. transmission crossed polars / Max. transmission parallel polars	Min. transmission parallel polars / Max. transmission crossed polars	Interference colour parallel polars
285	—	—	Yellow ($\frac{1}{2}\lambda$)	Red–blue I
295	—	—	Orange ($\frac{1}{2}\lambda$)	Blue
330	Deep yellow	—	Deep red ($\frac{1}{2}\lambda$)	Light blue
450	Orange	Blue (λ)	—	Light blue
485	Deep red	Blue–green (λ)	—	Blue–green
535	Red–blue I	Green (λ)	—	Green–yellow
575	Blue	Yellow (λ)	—	Yellow
590	Light blue	Orange (λ)	—	Deep yellow
660	Blue–green	Deep red (λ)	Blue ($1\frac{1}{2}\lambda$)	Deep yellow
730	Green–yellow	—	Blue–green ($1\frac{1}{2}\lambda$)	Orange
805	Yellow	—	Green ($1\frac{1}{2}\lambda$)	Deep red
855	Deep yellow	—	Yellow ($1\frac{1}{2}\lambda$)	Red–blue II
900	Orange	Blue (2λ)	Orange ($1\frac{1}{2}\lambda$)	Blue
970	Deep red	Blue–green (2λ)	Deep red ($1\frac{1}{2}\lambda$)	Blue–green
1075	Red–blue II	Green (2λ)	—	Green–yellow
1145	Blue	Yellow (2λ)	Blue ($2\frac{1}{2}\lambda$)	Deep yellow

Table 3

Interference colour	Minimum transmission	Maximum transmission
Red–blue	Yellow	—
Blue	Orange	—
Light blue	Red	(Blue)
Blue-green	—	Blue-green
Green	—	Dark green
Green-yellow	—	Green
Yellow	—	Yellow
Deep yellow	Blue	(Orange)
Orange	Blue-green	—
Red	Green	—

transmitted in terms of the associated spectral hue. It is clear from the table that when the analysing polar is rotated from the crossed to the parallel position, the red–blue junctions are shifted back along the wedge towards its narrow end by a distance equal to $\frac{1}{2}\lambda$, where λ = wavelength of yellow light. This shift, and the change in position of the intervening interference colours, can actually be seen occurring as the analyser is rotated, if a quarter wave plate is inserted into the optical path in the orthogonal position (with its slow direction parallel to the transmission axis of the polariser).

Table 2 throws some light on the genesis of interference colours. It can be seen that for the interference colours that correspond in hue to the colours of the more outlying parts of the spectrum, that is to say, violet, blue, light blue, deep yellow, orange, red, the main factor determining the colour is the wavelength minimally transmitted. Thus, for retardations up to 1150 nm, the interference colours blue, light blue, deep yellow, orange and red are associated with the withholding of orange, red, blue, blue-green and green spectral light respectively. With interference colours corresponding to coloured lights in the more central regions of the spectrum, the main determining factor is the wavelength maximally transmitted, so that the interference colours blue-green, green, green-yellow, yellow are associated respectively with maximum transmission of spectral blue-green, dark green, green and yellow. The interference colour (except in the case of yellow itself) is seen as yellower than the spectral light maximally transmitted, presumably because it contains a submaximal but nevertheless high proportion of yellow light, to which the eye is particularly sensitive. The relationships that hold between interference colours and transmission characters are set out in table 3.

It is also possible to extract from table 2 the pairs of 'complementary' interference colours obtained for any retardation by switching between crossed and parallel polars. These are blue/deep yellow; blue-green/orange; green/red; green-yellow/deep red; yellow/red–blue as shown in the 'colour pentagon' of fig. 2 (chapter 1). The colours blue, green, yellow, orange, deep red occupy the five angles of the pentagon, and the birefringence complementary of the colours at each angle is indicated by the colour represented by the opposite side.

Measurement of retardation

In order to make appropriate interference matches with McCollough colours, it is desirable to be able to measure the retardation of readily obtainable birefringent materials, such as samples of transparent adhesive tape. In general, wider tape is thicker, and so gives a greater retardation. When the retardations have been established, suitable layers can be built up in the addition or subtraction position to give retardations of $\frac{1}{2}\lambda$, λ, $1\frac{1}{2}\lambda$ or 2λ for any wavelength, and so produce the desired interference colour between crossed or parallel polars. The simplest way of measuring such retardations is by means of the quarter wave plate method of de Sénarmont, in which a $\frac{1}{4}\lambda$ plate is placed in the orthogonal position between the specimen and the analyser, and the analyser is rotated to produce extinction. If the polarising microscope has a Bertrand lens, this can be used to check the orthogonal position from the 'flash figure' formed between crossed polars. The principle of the $\frac{1}{4}\lambda$ plate method depends on the fact that light emerges from the specimen either linearly polarised in an orthogonal plane (retardations of 0, $\frac{1}{2}\lambda$, λ), or circularly polarised (retardations of $\frac{1}{4}\lambda$, $\frac{3}{4}\lambda$) or elliptically polarised (intermediate retardations). Linearly polarised light is not affected by the $\frac{1}{4}\lambda$ plate since it is in the orthogonal position, so that extinction is produced by rotating the analyser through angles of $0°$, $90°$, $180°$. Circularly polarised light of wavelength λ is converted by the $\frac{1}{4}\lambda$ plate into linearly polarised light in a diagonal plane, so that extinction is produced by rotating the analyser through angles of $45°$, $135°$. The $\frac{1}{4}\lambda$ plate can also be regarded as lying in a diagonal position relative to the fast and slow rays traversing the birefringent specimen, so that these components become circularly polarised in opposite directions, giving a linearly polarised resultant whose plane of polarisation can be detected by rotating the analyser. The retardation R is given by the formula $R = \lambda\theta/180$, where θ is the angle of rotation in degrees that is required to produce extinction. For a green light source ($\lambda = 546$ nm), the formula becomes $R = 3\theta$ nm.

It is often said that the $\frac{1}{4}\lambda$ plate method requires a monochromatic light source, but this is not so. If moderately birefringent material is examined by the method with a white light source the specimen is seen to darken to a deep blue. This becomes very apparent when the object being measured is the thin end of the quartz wedge. As the analyser is rotated the series of interference colours moves along the wedge as described in the previous section, until the first red–blue junction appears at the thin end. The de Sénarmont method can be used, therefore, with a white light source if the wave plate has a retardation of $\frac{1}{4}\lambda$ for yellow light. This will extinguish the yellow component of the white light, and the red–blue junction, i.e. the point at which the blue coloration just begins to change to red, is taken as the end-point. The colour-contrast obtained in this way actually gives a sharper end-point than the extinction obtained with monochromatic light.

With larger retardations, the end-point can be further improved by cutting down the amount of green in the incident light, with consequent intensification of the interference blue formed. This is achieved by using an interference red light source, e.g. from a $1\frac{1}{2}\lambda$ plate for green light between parallel polars as is used (chapter 3) for matching the red component of the McCollough effect. Such a wave plate can be made from adhesive tape with a retardation of 400 nm (i.e. $\frac{3}{4}\lambda$ for green light) applied lengthwise to either side of a microscope slide. To avoid having to adjust the wave plate precisely into the diagonal position between the polars, further pieces of the same tape can be applied diagonally to either side of the slide, one strip in the $+45°$ position and the other in the $-45°$ position. The compound plate so formed will yield an interference red in any position, not merely the diagonal, between parallel polars. If the tapes that are diagonal with respect to the slide are orthogonal with respect to the polars, all the birefringence is due to the two longitudinal pieces of tape. Their combined retardation $1\frac{1}{2}\lambda$ will cause green light to be held back by the second analysing polar. If the tapes that are diagonal with respect to the slide are also diagonal with respect to the polars, green light emerging from the first diagonal piece will be circularly polarised, and will remain circularly polarised on emerging from the two longitudinal pieces. This circularly polarised light will emerge from the second diagonal piece linearly polarised, and will be held back by the second polar. Interference red produced in this way and used in conjunction with a daylight filter as a light source emphasises the red–blue junction without distorting it (i.e. its position on a quartz wedge is not changed).

Maxwell's spot, Haidinger's brushes, coloured shadows
Certain visual phenomena resemble interference colours in that they are produced by the removal of some wavelengths from white light, and resemble McCollough colours in that this removal is achieved within the visual system. Maxwell's spot and Haidinger's brushes are termed entoptic phenomena, because the selective suppression of coloured light occurs within the eye. They are both believed to be due at least in part to the absorption of blue light by the pigment of the macula lutea in the foveal region of the retina. Maxwell's spot is seen at the fixation point when one looks at clouded sky through a cobalt blue filter. A dark spot begins to appear, rather slowly, and is probably caused partly by the absorption of blue light by macular pigment and partly by the greater susceptibility to fatigue of the blue mechanism of the fovea, where blue cones are scanty as compared with the peripheral retina. If, once Maxwell's spot has been seen, the filter is withdrawn about 30 cm from the eye, a bright turquoise or light blue spot appears at the fixation point, and returning the filter close to the eye then causes the dark spot to become more distinct. A similar manoeuvre with a purple filter (the Ilford micro 6 is particularly effective) produces a larger and brighter turquoise spot, which is replaced by a red spot when the filter is brought back to the eye. Moving the filter backwards and forwards causes the spots to alternate without fading.

More light can be thrown on the genesis of Maxwell's spot by selectively fatiguing different colour channels. If one looks at the clouded sky through an orange-red filter, the region of the fixation point soon comes to look brighter than the surround. Now replace the orange-red filter with a purple filter. A red spot is seen against a blue ground, as compared with the purple ground seen when the red receptors are not fatigued. These observations suggest that the red receptors of the fovea, unlike the blue receptors, are relatively resistant to fatigue as compared with those of the peripheral retina, where of course there are relatively few cones. When the filter is moved further from the eye, a turquoise spot appears as before. With prolonged fatigue of the red receptors, the fixation point no longer looks bright. When the orange-red filter is replaced with a purple filter, although the turquoise spot still appears when the filter is moved back, no red spot is seen with the filter close to the eye. Prolonged fatigue of the green mechanism does not produce a definite colour or intensity change at the fixation point. When the green filter is replaced with a purple filter, a red spot is seen against a purple ground, but little or no turquoise spot appears when the filter is moved back from the eye. One may infer from these experiments that the turquoise spot is an after-image caused by activation of the green mechanism and enhanced by red fatigue, and that it has the effect of itself promoting the red spot by causing fatigue of the green mechanism and activation of the red mechanism, especially in the partly dark-adapted retina.

Haidinger's brushes are seen, more rapidly than Maxwell's spot but in the same position, when the clouded sky is viewed through polarising material. The phenomenon is believed to be due to the pigment of the macula being orientated in such a way as to be radially dichroic, so that linearly polarised blue light is transmitted in the direction of its vibrations and absorbed at right angles to them. In consequence, the brushes proper point in a direction at right angles to the transmission axis of the polarising material; they are yellow in colour and appear to have diminished luminance because of the absorption of blue light. Between the arms of the brushes are light blue areas with an apparently enhanced brightness. Fatigue of the blue receptors with a blue filter causes a negative after-image of Maxwell's spot to be seen when the filter is removed, and when the after-image fades the yellow of the brushes is greatly enhanced. Fatiguing with green, on the other hand, causes the blue areas to appear a deeper and darker blue. To prevent the figure fading, it is necessary to rotate the polarising material repeatedly back and forth through 90°. If the polarising material has its transmission axis vertical or horizontal, the interposition of a $\frac{1}{4}\lambda$ birefringent plate for yellow light between it and the eye will cause the figure to reverse if the slow direction of the wave plate makes an angle of about 30° with the horizontal in an upwards and outwards direction, and to disappear if the slow direction is at right angles to this. These findings are consistent with a predominant orientation of the birefringent collagen of the cornea producing a resultant retardation of about 50 nm in the line of pull of the superior and inferior oblique muscles of the eye. The combined wave plate and cornea in the additive position are close to being a $\frac{1}{2}\lambda$ plate for blue light, and so they reverse the plane of polarisation and with it the orientation of the figure. In the subtractive position they approximate to a $\frac{1}{4}\lambda$ plate for blue light producing circularly polarised light which is then absorbed in all directions by the macula lutea. If a $\frac{1}{2}\lambda$ plate for yellow light is interposed, the effect is the opposite: the combined retardation of wave plate and cornea in the subtraction position is nearly a $\frac{1}{2}\lambda$ plate for blue light and so gives reversal, and in the addition position is a $\frac{3}{4}\lambda$ plate causing disappearance (Shute, 1974); see also *Scientific American*, December 1977 and *Vision Research* **18**, 1467.

The blue areas between Haidinger's brushes can be attributed to simultaneous colour contrast developing in a region where there is already a brightness contrast, and presumably result from inhibitory processes or from colour opponency operating in the visual system. Coloured shadows may be regarded as comparable phenomena. When unsaturated coloured light casts a shadow onto a white ground, that shadow if sufficiently intense, though still reflecting some light, will assume the complementary colour. Thus, yellow light will generate violet shadows, orange blue, red turquoise, magenta green, and vice versa. Some of these effects, which are extremely striking, are familiar to students of Impressionist painting. Like entoptic colours, shadow colours can be modified by fatiguing specific retinal receptors. Just as the Haidinger yellow is enhanced by previous exposure to the generating colour blue, so it is found that the intensity of shadow colours is markedly increased by adaptation to the various colours that generate them. Their hues can also be altered by adaptation to some other non-generating colours, in a way that can be predicted from the spectral sensitivities of retinal receptors. Thus, the yellow shadow produced by violet or blue light changes to green when the subject has previously adapted to red. Both the green shadow produced by magenta and the turquoise shadow produced by red become blue after adaptation to green light; this change can be compared with the deepening of the Haidinger blue that follows fatigue of the green receptors.

3

MEASURING METHODS

Previous methods

Science is measurement: or, according to Poincaré (1905), a concept that cannot be translated into numbers is, to a scientist, useless. So, in order to study the McCollough effect satisfactorily, it is essential to be able to quantify it, accurately, reproducibly, and in meaningful units. This can be done either by matching the phantom colours with similar known colours, or by a null method in which the phantom colours are cancelled by their complementaries, or by a combination of the two. The two best-known measuring methods that have been extensively used are that due to the MacKays (1973, 1975a) and that of Riggs and his school (Riggs et al., 1974; White, 1976). Both depend, partly or wholly, on neutralisation of the McCollough effect, and both require fairly complicated equipment. The MacKay method involves neutralisation of one McCollough colour component and matching of the other. It has the disadvantage that quantitation is in arbitrary units. A disturbing feature of the two approaches is that MacKay decay curves do not have the same shape as those obtained by the Riggs method.

The principle of the MacKay method is clearly illustrated in their 1975 paper, and I have to thank Professor Donald MacKay for his courtesy in demonstrating the apparatus to me personally. The testing and measuring procedure is as follows. The subject looks into a yellow-tinted illuminated box to see the test pattern, which has two windows lit from behind by diffused light from a projector. One window contains one element of the test pattern and is surrounded by the orthogonal contrasting pattern; the second window contains the other element of the test pattern, i.e. that surrounding the first window, and is itself surrounded by the pattern contained in the first window. In front of the projector is a mask transmitting a fixed amount of white light and a variable proportion of red to green light, produced by moving the boundary between a red and green filter across a slit in the mask with a pen-motor. The displacement of the red–green boundary from the centre of the slit is considered to be linearly related to the pen-motor current. The latter is taken to give a measure of the increase in red over green required to neutralise the green McCollough effect in one window and to match it with the red McCollough effect produced by its front-lit surround, and the increase in green over red required to neutralise the McCollough effect in the other window and to match it with the McCollough effect produced by its surround. The two together make up the total McCollough effect. If the subject tends to see either element of the test pattern as coloured before adaptation, this colour bias is measured by the same method and subtracted from the test readings.

The Riggs method, unlike that of the MacKays, is a purely null procedure. Neutralisation of the McCollough colours is achieved with complementary colours (green and magenta), and the amounts of each required to cause nullification are controlled with polarised light. The test pattern consists of a slide divided into four quadrants (later two areas only) covered by polaroid, so that white light from a projector traversing one component of the pattern in one pair of quadrants is linearly polarised, let us say horizontally in the direction of the pattern, while light traversing the orthogonal (vertical) component of the pattern in the other pair of quadrants is linearly polarised in the vertical direction. The light then passes through a central circular hole in a rotatable graduated disc. This hole is divided into three areas: a central clear slot (avoided in later versions) transmitting white light, and a segment on either side filled by a coloured filter, the one magenta and the other green. The coloured segments are covered by orthogonal polaroid, so that when the scale on the disc is in its central neutral position the transmission axis is at $45°$ to the transmission axes of the polaroid covering the test slide. Equal amounts of magenta and green light are then present in the horizontal and vertical components of the test pattern when these are projected onto a screen, so that, in the absence of a McCollough effect, these appear matched and approximately achromatic. Rotation of the disc through 45° in one direction will cause one component of the pattern, say the vertical, to receive only unsaturated magenta light, while the other, horizontal component receives only unsaturated green light. Rotation through 45° in the opposite direction will produce the opposite effects, and rotation through an amount less than 45° will produce magenta–green and green–magenta mixtures which can cancel the McCollough colours, so that the horizontal and vertical directional components of the test pattern, as seen projected onto the screen, again appear matched. The scale of measurement is calibrated in terms of the colorimetric purity of the light present in the pairs of quadrants in the test pattern, determined by measuring separately the relative luminances of the magenta, green and white components for each scale position. The strength of the McCollough effect is then expressed in terms of the change in colorimetric purity required to make the colour match.

Which method is to be preferred, that of the MacKays or that of Riggs? There is no doubt that the MacKay method gives precise and reproducible readings, and the decay curves obtained with it, when plotted on log–log co-ordinates, are impressively linear. By comparison, some of the earlier curves obtained by Riggs *et al.* (1974) and White (1976) seem decidedly ragged. Almost certainly this is because the colour match in the MacKay method provides a much more definite end-point than the achromatic match of the Riggs method. On the other hand, the mixture of colours used in the Riggs method is more exactly specified. The arbitrary units of strength, the use of a mixture of non-complementary colours to achieve cancellation and matching, and the consequent need to introduce an undetermined amount of yellow into the illumination of the surround pattern to balance the yellow of the red–green mix – these are unsatisfactory features of the MacKay procedure. Then there is the problem of the decay. It has already been mentioned that the MacKay and Riggs methods yield different-shaped decay curves. The MacKay curve is much steeper at first and flatter later than the Riggs curve, which in shape is very close to that obtained by the match interference method of measuring the strength of the McCollough effect (Shute, 1977*b*, *c*).

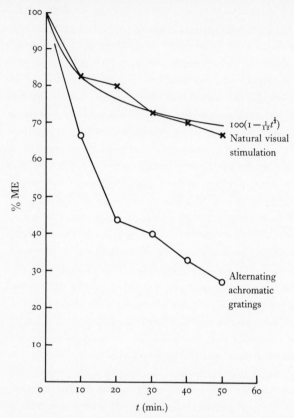

Fig. 4. Increase in ME decay rate produced by alternating achromatic gratings (Skowbo *et al.*, 1974). Normal decay rate given by $\% \text{ME} = 100(1 - \frac{1}{12}t^{1/3})$ where t = time in minutes after first test in a subject with a decay constant of $\frac{1}{12}$.

The match interference decay curve is also almost identical with the normal decay curve obtained by Skowbo *et al.* (1974), using another match method (fig. 4). Essentially the same results, then, have been obtained for the rate of decay of the McCollough effect from a pure null method and two pure match methods, all based on quite different principles. One is forced to conclude that the different type of curve obtained with the MacKay method results from some special feature of that method, and the most likely seems to be the combination of colour cancellation and matching leading to orthogonal test gratings being seen together against the same colour background. I have found that looking at orthogonal gratings through alternate red and green filters is an extremely effective way of rapidly expunging the McCollough effect. In one such experiment where red and green filters were alternated at 5 second intervals, a McCollough effect of initial strength ME = 62 (percentage suppression of green light required to match the red component) was reduced to ME = 38 in 5 minutes. Compare this with the normal decay occurring during a similar period, which would only bring down the strength to ME = 53 or 54. Put in another way, the decrement in ME strength after 5 minutes due to natural decay = 14 per cent of the initial strength, while the decrement after 5 minutes that results from looking at the test grating with alternating colours = 40 per cent of the initial strength. This latter figure is about double the decrement obtained by Skowbo *et al.* (1974) during the same period with achromatic gratings (fig. 4). These findings support the hypothesis that the rapid early decay that occurs with the MacKay measuring method is due to the matching procedure. The slow decay of later stages may result from relatively infrequent testing.

The match interference method

The apparatus for the match interference method of measuring the McCollough effect (Shute, 1977*b*) consists of an array of three mains-operated slide viewers free on a tray. The first viewer carries the coloured square-wave adapting gratings mounted side by side on a 5 cm × 5 cm slide. The bars and spaces of the adapting gratings are of equal width, and when observed at a distance of 30 cm through the viewer lens have a spatial frequency of 1 cycle per degree. The adapting colours are produced by Wratten filters nos. 58 (green: transmission peak at 530 nm) and 25 (orange-red: maximum transmission 610+ nm). Subjects view the adapting pattern for 5 minutes on a clockwork timer, spending 5 seconds on each grating before shifting their gaze to the other. They judge when to switch to the other grating by counting to themselves from 101 to 105. They choose a viewing distance that is comfortable for themselves (in my case, a hand's breadth with outstretched fingers from the viewer lens) and are instructed not to vary it, nor to turn their heads on one side. If they have reading glasses they are asked to wear them. Except for special purposes, amblyopes and colour-blind subjects are excluded. Subjects are told that they need not fixate, but can let their eyes move freely over the grating (the findings of Stromeyer and Mansfield (1970) and of Piggins and Leppmann (1973) suggest that it may be desirable to scan the grating); if they see the other grating out of the corners of their eyes, this does not matter. The ambient light is subdued. They should not have drunk tea or coffee for some hours previously. After adaptation is complete, subjects rest their eyes for 10 seconds before making the first measurement.

The achromatic test pattern is carried by the second slide viewer. It consists of a central grating in the form of an equilateral triangle, spatial frequency the same as that of the adapting slide, its bars orientated in the same direction as those of the green adapting grating, normally horizontal. Surrounding the central triangle is an orthogonal grating, with its bars in the same direction, therefore, as those of the red adapting grating. The luminance of the test slide is reduced by including a Wratten 0.3 neutral density filter. The third viewer, used for matching, contains a blank slide. Over the lens is fitted a circular stage graduated in degrees and carrying two pieces of polaroid with their axes of transmission parallel. Between the polars there is a rotating insert carrying a pointer which moves round the graduated scale. The insert is driven by a knob through a reducing gear, and is provided with a slot to take a 3×1 inch microscope slide. This slot holds a transparent birefringent $1\frac{1}{2}\lambda$ plate for green light ($\lambda = 535$ nm) with a retardation of 800 nm. Such a wave plate produces a red interference colour between parallel polars (see table 2), and the intensity of the colour increases from zero to a maximum as the angle between the slow direction of the wave plate and the transmission axis of the polars is increased from $0°$ to $45°$. A 1 inch square region of the wave plate is exposed for matching with the horizontal grating in the centre of the test slide. If the red component of the McCollough effect is matched after $c°$ of rotation, the percentage extinction of green light required to produce such a red $= 100 \sin^2 2c$, which can then be taken as a measure of the McCollough effect strength. The spectral composition of the match at a strength of ME $= 50$, i.e. when $c = 22\frac{1}{2}°$, is shown in fig. 5.

Matching, like adaptation, is carried out in subdued lighting conditions. Total darkness does not help the process. Subjects are

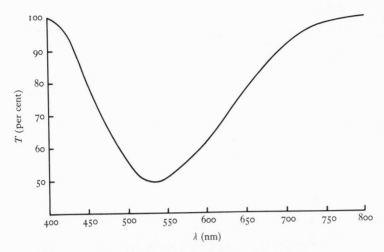

Fig. 5. Spectral transmittance of $1\frac{1}{2}\lambda$ plate for green light
(retardation = 800 nm) in $\pi/8$ position between parallel polars.
Calculated from $T = 100(1 - \frac{1}{2}\sin^2\frac{1}{2}\theta)$, where θ = phase
angle = $2\pi \times$ retardation/wavelength.

instructed to maintain the same distance from the test slide as
during adaptation. They must be particularly careful not to move
back from the viewer, since this will lead to a falsely high reading.
They should make the match quite rapidly, rotating once or twice
slightly above and below the eventual end-point, but not taking
more than 5 seconds in all. Prolonging the matching procedure does
not lead to greater accuracy. It is not usually necessary to take a
mean of several readings if the subject is familiar with the procedure.
With a little practice, experience shows that he can get reproducible
readings with an accuracy of $\frac{1}{2}°$. Because the interference colour
changes rapidly at the intensities commonly measured, the end-
point is usually settled upon with some confidence, and subjects
often comment on how well the interference colour reproduces the
McCollough colour that they see. The match is not impaired by
the reduced luminance of the interference system. This is due to
the two thicknesses of polaroid and was estimated photometrically
to be about 43 per cent. The addition of the 0.3 neutral density filter
to the test slide was decided upon empirically, because it was found
to make matching easier for most subjects. It is well known that
excessive brightness of the test pattern makes the McCollough

Table 4

$c°$	ME (%)	$c°$	ME (%)	$c°$	ME (%)
	0		27		76
1	0	16	28	31	78
	0		30		79
2	0	17	31	32	81
	1		33		82
3	1	18	35	33	83
	1		36		85
4	2	19	38	34	86
	2		40		87
5	3	20	41	35	88
	4		43		89
6	4	21	45	36	90
	5		47		91
7	6	22	48	37	92
	7		50		93
8	8	23	52	38	94
	9		53		95
9	10	24	55	39	96
	11		57		96
10	12	25	59	40	97
	13		60		98
11	14	26	62	41	98
	15		64		99
12	17	27	65	42	99
	18		67		99
13	19	28	69	43	100
	21		70		100
14	22	29	72	44	100
	24		73		100
15	25	30	75	45	100

effect harder to see. Within limits, varying the luminance is not crucial: subjects gave the same reading whether a neutral density filter was included or not. Remarkably enough, the subject while making the match is not aware of a luminance difference between the test slide and the interference colour. If, however, he turns his head through an angle of 45° so that the McCollough colours disappear, the test slide at once appears brighter.

When a value for $c°$, the number of degrees rotation required to

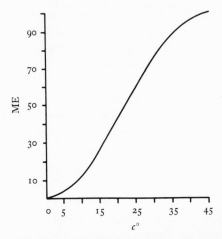

Fig. 6. Strength of McCollough effect expressed as percentage extinction of generating wavelength and given by $ME = 100 \sin^2 2c$ where $c° =$ angle of rotation of wave plate between parallel polars. $ME = 3\frac{1}{3}(c - 7\frac{1}{2})$ when c lies between $15°$ and $30°$.

produce a match, has been determined, the ME strength is read off from a $\sin^2$ table (table 4). Since c usually lies between $15°$ and $30°$ and a $\sin^2$ curve is virtually linear between these limits (see fig. 6), a useful approximation is given by

$$ME = 100 \sin^2 2c$$
$$= 3\frac{1}{3}(c - 7\frac{1}{2})$$

It is obvious from this equation that when $c = 15°$, $ME = 25$; when $c = 22\frac{1}{2}°$, $ME = 50$; and when $c = 30°$, $ME = 75$. An ME of 25 is very weak, and close to the lower limit of what can be detected. An ME of 50 is common in subjects who readily see a McCollough effect. With practice, values of 60–65 are often reached. An ME above 68 is rare. Subjective estimates of the strength of a McCollough effect are frequently erroneous, even in experienced observers. Naive subjects often report the effect as being 'very faint', although the measured strength may be 50. They are then amazed to be told that the colour they see is the equivalent of removing half the green content of white light.

Note that in assessing the strength of the McCollough effect, any initial colour bias that may be seen on the test pattern before adaptation is not added to or subtracted from the measured value. For most purposes, this is not a desirable practice. In the first place, there is reason to believe that subthreshold McCollough effects can be present that are too small to measure. More importantly, however, the subsequent behaviour of a McCollough effect depends upon its initial strength no matter how that strength is arrived at; that is to say, whether it is built up on a previous McCollough effect of the same type or not. Consequently, it only becomes necessary to take account of a pre-adaptation level if some parameter, such as luminance of the adapting pattern, is being investigated in relation to the McCollough effect strength eventually achieved.

Making wave plates

Excellent plastic $1\frac{1}{2}\lambda$ plates for green light, suitable for measuring the strength of McCollough effects by the match interference method, can be obtained from Mr Bassett, James Swift and Son Ltd, Joule Road, Basingstoke, England. The reader may like, however, to construct wave plates for himself, and so increase the range of interference colours available to him. I have made and routinely used wave plates by combining, in the addition or subtraction position as appropriate, various widths and so various thicknesses of birefringent transparent adhesive tape applied to glass slides. 'Caribonum polytape' proved to be very suitable. The retardations of the various samples of tape were measured by the $\frac{1}{4}$ wave plate method of de Sénarmont (see chapter 2) or with a Babinet variable compensator, and wave plates were constructed as in table 5.

Unfortunately different reels of the same widths of tape have different retardations, so this table must be taken as a guide only. When a wave plate made in this way is set between parallel polars, the intensity of the lights transmitted is determined partly by its position relative to the transmission axis of the polars and partly by its phase angle.

If $c° =$ angle between slow direction of wave plate and transmission axis of polars, and $\theta° =$ phase angle of wave plate $= (R/\lambda) \times 360°$ where $R =$ retardation of wave plate and $\lambda =$ wavelength of light, then

$$\text{percentage transmission} = 100(1 - \sin 2c \sin^2 \tfrac{1}{2}\theta)$$

When $c = 22\frac{1}{2}°$, $\sin^2 2c = \frac{1}{2}$; therefore

Table 5 *Construction of wave plates from adhesive tape for use with parallel polars*

λ (nm)	Wave plates λ	Adhesive tape (inches)	Interference colour
455	455	$1\frac{1}{2}+\frac{1}{2}$	Light blue
495	495	$1+$ two $\times \frac{1}{2}$	Blue-green
525	525	Two $\times 1\frac{1}{2}+\frac{1}{2}-1$	Green-yellow
580	580	Two $\times 1\frac{1}{2}-\frac{1}{2}$	Yellow II
590	590	Two $\times \frac{3}{4}+\frac{1}{2}$	Deep yellow
	$1\frac{1}{2}\lambda$		
440	660	Two $\times 1+\frac{1}{2}$	Deep yellow
490	735	$1+\frac{3}{4}+$ two $\times \frac{1}{2}$	Orange
535	800	Two $\times 1\frac{1}{2}+\frac{1}{2}$	Deep red
575	860	$1\frac{1}{2}+1+\frac{3}{4}$	Red–blue II
600	900	Two $\times 1+\frac{3}{4}+\frac{1}{2}$	Blue
640	960	Two $\times 1\frac{1}{2}+1$	Blue-green
	2λ		
515	1030	Two $\times 1+$ two $\times \frac{3}{4}$	Green
535	1065	Three $\times 1+\frac{3}{4}$	Green-yellow
575	1145	Three $\times 1\frac{1}{2}+\frac{1}{2}$	Yellow III

Retardations of adhesive tape: $1\frac{1}{2}$ in., 345; 1 in., 275; $\frac{3}{4}$ in., 240; $\frac{1}{2}$ in., 110.

$$\text{percentage transmission} = 100(1-\tfrac{1}{2}\sin^2\tfrac{1}{2}\theta)$$

This is the formula used to calculate the transmittance of the $1\frac{1}{2}\lambda$ plate for green light (fig. 5). When $R = \frac{1}{2}\lambda$ or $1\frac{1}{2}\lambda$, $\sin^2\frac{1}{2}\theta = 1$; therefore

$$\text{percentage transmission} = 100(1-\sin^2 2c)$$
$$= 100\cos^2 2c$$

So, when a $\frac{1}{2}\lambda$ or $1\frac{1}{2}\lambda$ plate is rotated between parallel polars, the diminution in light intensity obeys a cosine^2 law (fig. 7).
Similarly,

$$\text{percentage extinction} = 100\sin^2 2c \sin^2\tfrac{1}{2}\theta$$

When $R = \frac{1}{2}\lambda$ or $1\frac{1}{2}\lambda$, $\sin^2\frac{1}{2}\theta = 1$; therefore

$$\text{percentage extinction} = 100\sin^2 2c$$

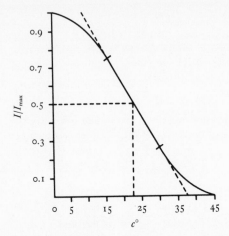

Fig. 7. Diminution in light intensity produced by rotating $\frac{1}{2}\lambda$ or $1\frac{1}{2}\lambda$ plate between parallel polars, given by $I/I_{max} = \cos^2 2c$, where c = angle of rotation. Intensity halved at $22\frac{1}{2}°$, curve linear between $15°$ and $30°$.

which is the formula from which the strength of the McCollough effect is calculated.

In general, $1\frac{1}{2}\lambda$ plates are most satisfactory for measuring the strength of McCollough colours, since the 2nd Order interference colours that they generate are particularly clear, and the calculation is simple. On the other hand, λ plates can also be used, as in the following example. The McCollough colour generated by blue light (Wratten filter no. 47B: $\lambda = 430$ nm) was matched by a λ plate for orange light, $R = 590$ nm, rotated through an angle $c = 25°$

$$ME = 100 \sin^2 2c \sin^2 \tfrac{1}{2}\theta, \quad \text{where} \quad \theta = \tfrac{590}{430} \times 360°$$
$$= 100 \sin^2 50° \sin^2 67°$$
$$= 50$$

Unlike other McCollough colours, a phantom green cannot be quantified in terms of the percentage extinction of the generating wavelength, since green cannot be formed by destructive interference (see table 2). The green generated by adaptation to red in the standard method can be matched, however, with a 2λ plate for deep green.

Evaluation of the method

Results obtained with the match interference method of quantifying the McCollough effect agree well with those obtained by most other methods. It appears also to have some real merits of its own. The apparatus is simple and cheap to make, and very transportable. Subjects find it easy to use, and are not intimidated by it. It is sensitive, and gives reproducible results. It measures in meaningful units. It is easily modified for use with different adapting patterns and colours. The experimenter has the advantage of being able to view an almost exact replica of the phantom colour that the subject sees. The way in which the interference colour is formed, through subtotal extinction of a particular wavelength with lesser extinction of adjacent wavelengths, may well mimic inhibitory processes that actually occur in the visual system during the production of the McCollough effect. Such inhibitory processes could account for the apparent reduction of luminance produced by the phantom colours in the test slide.

4

STRENGTH OF THE McCOLLOUGH EFFECT

General considerations

One advantage that stems from the portability of the equipment used for quantifying the McCollough effect by the match interference method is that it is possible to make the measurements not in the context of a laboratory experiment but as part of the changing circumstances of everyday life. The rate of decay of the McCollough effect is determined by the initial strength according to the formula presented and discussed in chapter 6 so that, for any particular subject at a given time after first testing, there is an expected strength that can be predicted, other things being equal, with a high level of confidence. By altering the environment in various ways, one can look for influences on the McCollough effect that cause either depression associated with more rapid decay or elevation associated with slower decay. Such influences, once they have been established must be avoided during testing when the possible effect of another environmental factor is being looked for, or if a typical decay curve is to be obtained.

The four commonest factors that I have found to influence the McCollough effect are coffee (or tea), muscular activity, stress and fatigue. The first three tend to depress the McCollough effect or accelerate its decay, and the last has the opposite actions. They are discussed in detail in subsequent chapters.

The most dramatic example of the effect of fatigue I have seen was in an amblyopic subject (see also chapter 5). This subject, a female student with a history of squint, had impaired vision in one eye such that the adapting and test gratings appeared extremely blurred when viewed with that eye alone. She was also myopic. She adapted in the usual way, and on testing monocularly with the bad eye first, the ME strength in that eye was 70, while the ME strength in the good eye was 38. She was as surprised as I then was by the quite unusual strength of the McCollough effect in the amblyopic eye. When retested a week later, the ME strength was 35 in each eye. On being questioned as to what might have been different on the two occasions to account for the discrepancy, she confessed that at the first testing she was excessively tired, having had scarcely any sleep the night before. My research student Mr Amure has informed me that after a night without sleep his McCollough effect was very high and virtually failed to decay. I have consistently found that McCollough effects induced in myself late at night are higher than those induced in the morning. Curiously, MacKay and MacKay (1975b, 1977) have reported that they have found the strength to be often higher in the morning than the night before. Possibly there is some difference here in the degree of fatigue before retiring and on waking.

The effects of fatigue on the one hand, and stimulating factors such as coffee, muscular activity and stress on the other, would appear to favour the hypothesis that the McCollough effect is primarily an inhibitory phenomenon involving the depression of a specific colour channel but influenced by conditions that cause a general depression or elevation of nervous activity in the brain. If this is so, the strength of the McCollough effect may in part reflect levels of arousal. It is often said that arousal levels show diurnal variation, being greatest about noon and less at the beginning and end of the day. I have not detected diurnal rhythms in the McCollough effect other than what can be attributed to different degrees of tiredness, and to the taking of stimulating drinks which in many subjects is greatest in the morning.

Methods of reducing initial strength

Apart from the taking of coffee, there are four main ways in which the initial strength of the McCollough effect can be reduced, through varying the parameters of the adapting and test stimuli. First, a lack of conformity may be introduced between the adapting and test gratings, either an angular or a size discrepancy: with adapting gratings of a relatively low spatial frequency, widening the spaces and narrowing the bars of the test gratings reduces the intensity of the induced colours. Secondly, desaturating the adapting colours has a similar effect. When the McCollough effect is demonstrated to a mass audience, it is convenient to use a large screen and to project adapting gratings made from photographic film, since gelatine filters are liable to melt. It is impossible to get highly saturated colours in this way, and although most of the audience will be able to see McCollough colours, there may be some who have to re-adapt with more saturated colours to get a measurable effect. Thirdly, the adaptation time may be shortened. Even naive subjects usually develop measurable McCollough effects after 3–5 minutes, although a few may require longer. Practised subjects may develop McCollough effects after little more than a glance, and for this reason, if a planned low intensity effect is required, it is better to adopt the fourth method, namely, reduced adaptation luminance.

White (1976) measured the strength and decay of the McCollough effect in two subjects adapting at three different luminances. As would be expected lower luminances produced lower strengths, but his plots show no constant relationship between the two. In one subject, himself, reduction of luminance to 12 per cent of the highest luminance used (30 foot lamberts) reduced the McCollough effect strength by only 20 per cent, whereas in the other subject the same reduction in luminance reduced the McCollough effect strength by 70 per cent.

I have investigated the relationship between adaptation luminance and McCollough effect strength using polarised light (Shute, 1977c). The light was made to pass through two strips of polaroid, one of which could be rotated with respect to the other so that the angle between the two transmission axes could be varied and measured. If the angle between the transmission axis of the polars $= \phi°$, then the percentage intensity loss due to the obliquity of the polars $= 100 \sin^2 \phi$. The intensity loss due to the two thicknesses of polaroid with axes of transmission parallel ($\phi = 0°$) was measured photometrically and taken to be 45 per cent. If the light intensity without the intervention of polars is 100, then the reduction in intensity $\% I$ due to setting the polars at various angles ϕ is shown in table 6.

During the early stages of my investigations I was repeatedly

Table 6

Angle between transmission areas of polars (ϕ)	90°	75°	60°	45°	30°	0°
Percentage of intensity without polars (% I)	0	3	11	$22\frac{1}{2}$	34	45

Table 7

Percentage of intensity without polars (% I)	0	11	$22\frac{1}{2}$	34	45	100
McCollough effect strength (ME)	0	35	41	43	45	50

Table 8

Percentage of intensity without polars (% I)	0	3	11	100
McCollough effect strength (ME)	0	33	41	60

obtaining with normal adaptation, i.e. without the intervention of polars, an initial McCollough effect strength of $ME_0 = 50$. I then inserted polars at various angles to reduce the adapting luminance (% I) as in table 6, and obtained values for the ME as in table 7. Using these figures I plotted ME against % I on log–log co-ordinates and obtained a straight line with a gradient of 1/6. The intercept on the ordinate was 24. It was therefore possible to write the equation

$$ME = 24(\% I)^{1/6} \quad \text{when} \quad ME_0 = 50$$

At a later date when my initial ME strength was habitually $ME_0 = 60$, I remeasured the ME for $\phi = 75°$ and $\phi = 60°$, i.e. for values of % $I = 3$ and % $I = 11$ (table 6), and obtained values for the ME as in table 8. Again, the log–log plot of ME against % I was linear with a gradient of 1/6. The intercept was 28, yielding the equation

$$ME = 28(\% \, I)^{1/6} \quad \text{when} \quad ME_0 = 60$$

On the assumption that the relationship between ME and $\% \, I$ is determined by other values of ME_0 in the same manner, we can generalise the equations as follows

$$ME = \tfrac{7}{15}ME_0(\% \, I)^{1/6}$$

or

$$\frac{ME}{ME_0} = \tfrac{7}{15}(\% \, I)^{1/6}$$

Returning to the results of White (1976), it is interesting that the values he obtained on himself for McCollough effect strengths when $\% \, I = 100$ (30 ft L) and $\% \, I = 12.3$ (3.7 ft L) approximately fit the above equation. The curves relating ME to $\% \, I$ when $ME_0 = 50$ and when $ME_0 = 60$ are shown in fig. 8.

   There are some corollaries of the relationship between adaptation luminance and McCollough effect strength. First, increasing the luminance further has relatively little influence on the McCollough effect: if the same relationship held, the adapting luminance would have to be increased over fifty times to raise the ME from 50 to 100. Secondly, very substantial drops in luminance are required to produce a marked effect on the ME: for instance, a 98 per cent reduction in luminance is required to halve the ME strength. This means that the McCollough effect mechanism is operative over a wide range of luminances such as one might meet in everyday life. Thirdly, by controlling the adaptation luminance it is possible to plan in advance to obtain a particular strength of the McCollough effect. This proved particularly useful in working out the relationship between the rate of decay of the McCollough effect and its initial strength (chapter 6). Occasionally, however, the MEs actually obtained were higher than their predicted values. This happened when a McCollough effect was induced rather soon, i.e. not more than a day after a previous induction, or when a previous McCollough effect had not been expunged by regular testing. There can be little doubt that these high values were due to the presences of residual MEs, in themselves below the threshold of measurement. Controlling the luminance of a subsequent induction provides a method of detecting and even quantifying such subliminal MEs. Thus, when the initial ME produced by adapting without polars

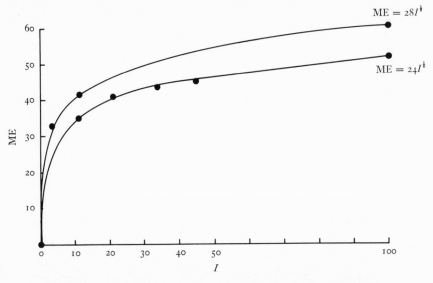

Fig. 8. ME and adapting luminance, reduced with rotating polars. If
$\% I$ = percentage of intensity without polars, ME_0 = ME strength
without polars, then reduced ME strength is given by
$ME = \frac{7}{15} ME_0 \, I^{1/6}$.

is 60, and the polars are set at angles of $60°$ with a view to producing
an ME of 41, the actual ME strength attained may be, say 55. This
will indicate the presence of a residual ME of 14, which on its own
is too small to measure.

Effects of coloured lights

The strength and decay of the red and green components of the
McCollough effect can be modified by flooding the eyes with red
or green light. First it is worth describing the effect of a red (acetate)
filter transmitting only red, and some orange and yellow light, on
low colour intensities such as those of coloured objects seen by
reflected light. Blue and green objects appear black. This is because
blue objects reflect no yellow or red light, and the amount of yellow
light reflected by green objects that is able to pass the filter is not
sufficient to activate the retinal receptors. Yellow objects, which
reflect green and orange light as well as yellow, appear whitish as
a result of the removal of the green and partial removal of the
orange. Red objects appear yellow, or colourless if there is little

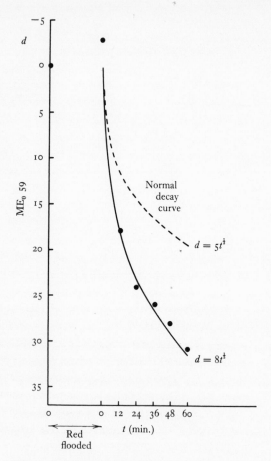

Fig. 9. Increase in ME decay rate produced by wearing red shield for 36 minutes after first test. d = decrement below initial strength ME_0.

content of yellow in the light reflected by them. This is because of the relative insensitivity of the retina to red: the amount of red light reflected by the object and transmitted by the filter is below threshold level.

Covering the eyes with a red filter affects the McCollough effect in different ways during the wearing of the filter and after the filter is removed. While the filter is being worn, there is no activation of the green colour channel in the visual system and there is diminished absolute activation of the red channel, since the amount of red light transmitted by the filter is rather less than the red

Table 9 *Effect of red flooding* (*exclusion of green*)

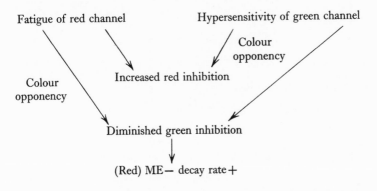

Fatigue of red channel   Hypersensitivity of green channel

Colour opponency

Increased red inhibition

Colour opponency

Diminished green inhibition

(Red) ME— decay rate+

component of white light. There will, of course, be increased relative activation of the red channel as compared with the green, the colour opponency from the latter will have been removed. In consequence, during this period inhibition of green due to a previously established McCollough effect is maintained or increased. This was seen when the ME was measured immediately before and after flooding the eyes with red for 36 minutes: the ME rose from an initial value of $ME_0 = 59$ by three points to 62 (fig. 9).

When the red filter is removed the green channel, which has become hypersensitive from disuse, is activated and the inhibition of green rapidly diminishes. In consequence the ME (i.e. the red component of the McCollough effect) decays more rapidly and the values obtained on measurement fall (fig. 9). The inhibition of red, on the other hand, will be increased, partly on account of relative fatigue of the red channel, partly in response to hyperactivity of the green channel through a colour opponency mechanism. The factors probably operating after the eyes have been flooded with red, i.e. after green light has been excluded, are illustrated in table 9.

A similar acceleration of ME decay occurs when the eyes are flooded with red light for 36 minutes before adaptation (fig. 10). This procedure enhances the green component and in no way depresses the initial red component of the McCollough effect.

The effect of flooding the eyes with green light or of excluding red light is not quite the opposite of what occurs when they are flooded with red or when green is excluded. If red is excluded with

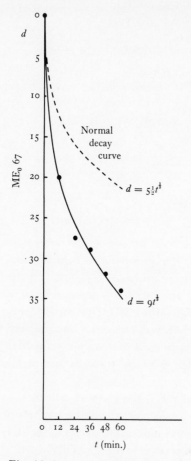

Fig. 10. Increase in ME decay rate produced by wearing red shield for 36 minutes before adaptation.

Table 10 *Effect of red exclusion* (*excess of green*)

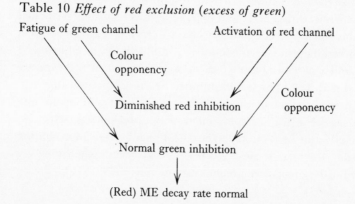

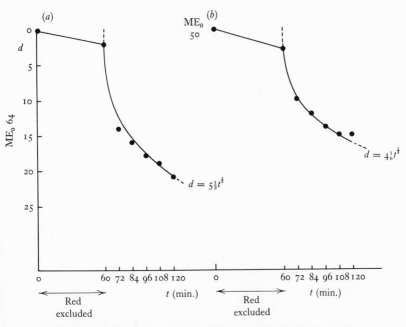

Fig. 11. Effect of excluding red from both eyes for 60 minutes after first test (two experiments, different initial strengths). Decay partially arrested during red exclusion, subsequent decay rate normal.

a green filter or through wearing anti-laser glasses containing interference filters that exclude all and only orange and red light, there is a small drop in ME strength while the filters are being worn, but much less than the normal decay that would occur during that period. After the filters are removed, ME decay occurs at the normal rate (fig. 11).

What is the reason for this difference? One may suppose that during the wearing of the filters the green channel is facilitated by the removal of red opponency so that decay of the ME is arrested, but that when the filters are removed, the return of colour opponency does not result in increased inhibition of green in the green channel, but causes the inhibition of green to revert to normal, so that ME decay proceeds at the usual rate (table 10). If the eyes are flooded with green light for 10 minutes before adaptation, a strong red component of the McCollough effect is formed but no green components can be seen.

Stereopsis and the McCollough effect

Random dot stereographic pairs (Julesz, 1971) are formed from
identical dot patterns with a central area in one stereogram
displaced horizontally either in an inwards direction towards the
other stereogram, or in an outwards direction away from it. An
illusion of depth is created: the central area appears nearer to the
observer if the displacement has been inwards, and further away
if the displacement has been outwards. The reason for this lies in
the retinal disparity which occurs between the two eyes when the
observer views two objects that are more or less directly ahead and
different distances away. The images of the nearer object are more
laterally placed on the retinae than those of the further object. For
this reason the brain learns to interpret lateral retinal displacement
as a sign of nearness. Because of the inversion produced by the
lenses of the two eyes, an inwards displacement of the central area
in random dot stereograms causes an outwards displacement or
discrepancy on the retinae, so that when the stereo pairs are fused
the central area is interpreted as being closer to the observer. Two
other interesting visual illusions are associated with the illusion of
depth. First there is an illusion of parallax. If the observer moves
his head from side to side, the apparently nearer of the two
patterns, centre or surround according to how the stereo pairs are
arranged, seems to move with respect to the pattern that appears
further off. The brain is deceived because of the association that
normally occurs between distance and parallax. If the observer
concentrates on the relative positions of two random dots, one in
the centre and one in the surround, he sees that there is actually
no parallax. Secondly there is an illusion of size. If the central area
is displaced so as to appear closer to the observer, it seems to be
smaller in size. This often causes some surprise, since observers
think that a nearer object should appear larger, not smaller. The
reason for the illusion is simple. Since the central area is actually
still in the same plane as the surround, the angle that it subtends
at the eye is not changed. Nearer objects subtending a given angle
at the eye are smaller than further objects subtending the same
angle. Therefore the brain interprets the apparently nearer object
as being smaller.

Julesz (1971) describes some unsuccessful experiments to determine whether the McCollough effect is established at a higher or

lower level than stereopsis in the central nervous system. The idea was to discover whether phantom colours could aid or interfere with fusion, but the colour saturation turned out to be too weak to produce any measurable effect. I reversed the experiment, to see whether Julesz type stereo pairs consisting of small orthogonal gratings instead of random dots produced any change in the strength of the McCollough effect after stereopsis was established. I found that the creation of a depth illusion did not alter the strength of a McCollough effect.

Because of the coarseness of the grain of the pattern, it takes observers much longer, often 20–30 seconds, to establish stereopsis when the stereograms are made from mini-gratings rather than dots. Ramachandran (1976) has commented that the time required to develop stereopsis improves with practice, but has found that the acquisition of this skill is specific to the area of retina involved, since viewing at a different angle causes the stereopsis time to lengthen again. This type of localised learning suggests a parallel with the McCollough effect, where the effective stimulus is normally the direction of the grating as registered at the fovea. A McCollough effect set up at the fovea by looking directly at the adapting gratings is not evoked when the head is turned to one side to involve only the peripheral retina (see Stromeyer, 1972b).

Stereopsis is conveniently tested by projecting superimposed random dot stereo pairs with light polarised in orthogonal planes. The screen is then viewed through orthogonally orientated polaroid spectacles. This has proved a useful method of picking out amblyopic subjects, i.e. those with defective vision in one eye, usually associated with a history of squint. Such subjects lack stereopsis. Some features of the McCollough effect in amblyopes are presented and discussed in chapter 5.

5

MONOCULAR, INTEROCULAR AND NON-REDUNDANT EFFECTS

Monocular and interocular effects of red and green lights
When one eye only is subjected to red or green light, ocular interaction occurs so that the strength and decay of a previously established McCollough effect is modified in the other eye. In an experiment when one eye was covered with a red filter for 36 minutes immediately after the first test which registered a McCollough effect strength of $ME_0 = 64$, the McCollough effect in the uncovered contralateral eye decayed more rapidly than the normal rate for this initial strength, which is given by $d = 5\frac{1}{3}t^{1/3}$, where d is the decrement below the initial strength and t is the time in minutes (see chapter 6). When after 36 minutes the red filter was removed, the decay of the McCollough effect was almost totally arrested in the contralateral eye for the next hour (fig. 12(a)). By contrast, the ME in the eye that had been covered began to decay rapidly, at a rate resembling that of the contralateral eye earlier, and also that seen after both eyes have been red flooded (chapter 4, fig. 9). There was, therefore, a complete dissociation between the decay rates of the two eyes: after removal of the filters the previously covered eye was producing a rapid decay while the ME in the contralateral eye that had been uncovered throughout was decaying scarcely at all. The mechanisms possibly accounting for the responses of the contralateral eye to monocular red flooding are set out in table 11.

In another experiment, excluding red from one eye with anti-laser glasses for a similar time of 36 minutes after recording a

Table 11 *Effect of monocular red flooding on contralateral eye*

(*a*) During flooding: ME decay +

Depression of red channel

| Colour opponency
↓

Activation of green channel

|
↓

Diminished green inhibition

(*b*) After flooding: ME decay −

Activation of red channel

| Colour opponency
↓

Depression of green channel

|
↓

Increased green inhibition

McCollough effect initial strength of $ME_0 = 59$ produced quite different results. The McCollough effect in the uncovered contra-lateral eye during this period began by increasing in strength but then fell rapidly (fig. 12(*b*)), so that by the time the interference filter was removed the decay rate was similar to that seen after red flooding. After removal of the filter the ME in the previously covered eye decayed at a normal rate, so that once again there was dissociation between the two eyes. Possible mechanisms are shown in table 12.

The results of these experiments on ocular interaction can be summed up as follows. Excess of green to one eye produces

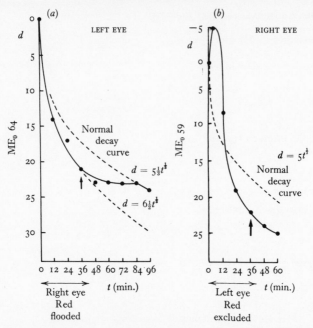

Fig. 12. Effects on contralateral ME decay of (a) wearing red shield over one eye and (b) excluding red from one eye for 36 minutes after first test.

simultaneous and subsequent responses in the other eye as though it were receiving an excess of red light. Excess of red to one eye produces simultaneous and subsequent responses in the other eye which are the reverse of those produced by excess green.

Non-redundant binocular McCollough effects

To set up a McCollough effect it is not necessary that the adapting stimulus should consist of two contrasting patterns and two colours. A single pattern and a single colour, presented simultaneously or alternately, can be enough. I shall call McCollough effects produced by a single pattern and single colour *non-redundant*, and those produced by two patterns and two colours *redundant*. Non-redundant and redundant McCollough effects can be binocular or dichoptic: in the latter case, one eye is pattern stimulated and the other eye is colour stimulated. Redundant dichoptic effects have been studied by MacKay and MacKay (1973, 1975a).

Table 12 *Effect of monocular red exclusion on contralateral eye*

(*a*) Initially during exclusion: ME decay −

Activation of red channel

| Colour opponency
↓

Depression of green channel

|
↓

Increased green inhibition

(*b*) Followed by: ME decay +

Depression of red channel

| Colour opponency
↓

Activation of green channel

|
↓

Diminished green inhibition

Stromeyer (1969) described semi-redundant binocular McCollough effects produced by a pattern plus colour alternating with an achromatic orthogonal pattern, and non-redundant binocular effects produced by a pattern plus colour alternating with a period of darkness of equal duration. Murch and Hirsch (1972) alternated pattern and colour to produce non-redundant binocular after-effects.

I have studied and measured two types of non-redundant binocular McCollough effect, that produced by an achromatic grating alternating with the adapting colour green, and that produced by grating plus green alternating with white light (fig. 13). The sequence in the second type differs from that of Stromeyer (1969) in that the use of alternating white light rather than darkness

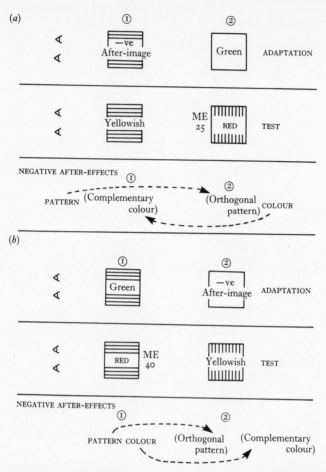

Fig. 13. Binocular non-redundant MEs: (*a*) alternation of *one* grating with *one* colour; (*b*) alternation of *one* grating plus colour with white light. For further description, see text.

permits the adapting colour to generate a negative after-image, which can itself then act as an adapting colour to produce a McCollough effect (Murch and Hirsch, 1972). The sequence in the first type of non-redundant binocular McCollough effect (fig. 13(*a*)) was as adopted by Murch and Hirsch. Green alternating with an achromatic horizontal grating causes a magenta or purplish negative after-image to be superimposed on that grating. When the test pattern is viewed, a phantom red is seen associated with the vertical grating, whereas the horizontal grating appears yellowish. *Pace* Murch and Hirsch, a true McCollough green, such as would be produced by adapting to a grating plus red, is not seen. The yellowish colour is, however, the expected response to the purplish colour of the negative after-image produced by green (see table 1). The phantom red was measured and found to have a strength of $ME = 25$. In this experiment the system is behaving as if an orthogonal pattern were presented in conjunction with the adapting colour, but the ME is much weaker than it would have been if the orthogonal grating had actually been present.

When during adaptation the horizontal grating and the adapting colour green are presented simultaneously so as to alternate with an unpatterned purplish negative after-image, it is the horizontal component of the test pattern that now develops a phantom red, and the vertical component that is yellowish (fig. 13(*b*)). The colour and pattern presented to the stimulated eye induce in the unstimulated eye the complementary colour, actually present as the negative after-image, and the effect of the orthogonal pattern, although this is not in fact seen. The ME strength is now 40, i.e. higher than when the adapting colour alternated with the pattern. Stronger non-redundant MEs are produced when pattern and colour are simultaneous than when they alternate.

Non-redundant dichoptic effects

In view of the ocular interactions produced by red and green described in chapter 4 I decided to investigate the nature and strengths of non-redundant dichoptic McCollough effects in the various possible combinations of adapting stimuli. Some of the results have been briefly reported already (Shute, 1977*d*). In the following analysis of experiments carried out on myself, the pattern-stimulated eye, which was sometimes the left and sometimes the right, will be referred to as 'eye A' and the colour-stimulated eye as 'eye B'. Rather different results were obtained when green was the adapting colour (fig. 14) from those which were obtained when red was the adapting colour (fig. 15). When, during adaptation, eye A saw the pattern, a horizontal grating, and eye B saw the colour, green, alternately so that eye B saw the negative after-image of green simultaneously with the pattern seen by eye A it was found at test that eye A saw a weak red McCollough effect, strength ME = 25, associated with the horizontal grating (fig. 14(*a*)). The induced colour associated with the vertical grating was yellowish, and eye B did not detect any colour associated with the test pattern. Comparing this result with the non-redundant binocular McCollough effect (fig. 13), we see that alternation of patterns with green has again produced a weak ME, but now the McCollough effect is reversed, that is to say the phantom red is associated with the horizontal part of the test pattern, not the vertical part. The pattern-stimulated eye behaves as if it had seen, simultaneously with the pattern, the colour seen by the colour-stimulated eye during the intervening period when the pattern-stimulated eye was not receiving a pattern stimulus. In other words, the adapting colour green presented to one eye subsequently induces the effects of green in the other (pattern-stimulated) eye (Shute, 1977c). It is possible that an important factor in generating the red McCollough effect in the pattern-stimulated eye is the negative after-image which develops, simultaneously with that pattern, in the colour-stimulated eye. The ocular interactions presumed to be involved are illustrated in fig. 14(*a*).

When, during adaptation, eye A saw the horizontal grating and eye B saw green simultaneously, it was found at test that the red McCollough effect was again associated with the horizontal part of the pattern, but this time in eye B instead of in eye A (fig. 14(*b*)). The strength was considerably greater (ME = 40). Again comparing with the non-redundant binocular effects (fig. 13), we note that a stronger ME is obtained when green is presented simultaneously with the adapting grating than when it alternates. Eye A saw a greenish colour associated with the horizontal part of the test pattern. In this experiment the McCollough effect is not reversed, that is to say the phantom red is associated with the horizontal pattern which was presented during adaptation simultaneously with the green, as in binocular viewing.

The colour-stimulated eye behaves as if it had seen, simultaneously with the colour, the pattern seen by the pattern-stimulated eye (fig. 14(*b*)). In other words, the adapting pattern presented to one eye *simultaneously* induces the effects of that pattern in the other (colour-stimulated) eye (Shute, 1977c).

The results of green induction of non-redundant dichoptic McCollough effects can be summarised as follows. A red after-effect

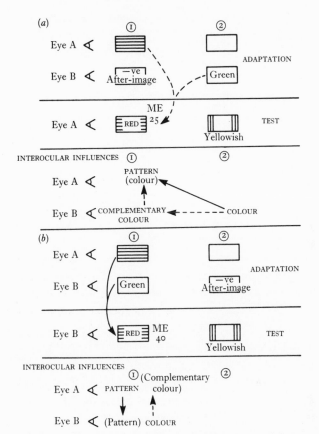

Fig. 14. Dichoptic non-redundant MEs: green induction. (a) Pattern alternating with colour; (b) pattern simultaneous with colour. Eye A pattern stimulated, eye B colour stimulated.

is produced in association with the portion of the test pattern that corresponds to the adapting pattern, whether the adapting colour is presented simultaneously with the adapting colour or alternately. In the latter case the red McCollough effect is seen only by the pattern-stimulated eye, and is weak; in the former case the red McCollough effect is seen only by the colour-stimulated eye, and is stronger. In the adaptation phase, colour presented to one eye produces simultaneous effects in the other eye as if that eye were seeing the complementary colour, whereas the effects of pattern transfer directly to the opposite eye.

The non-redundant dichoptic McCollough effects obtained

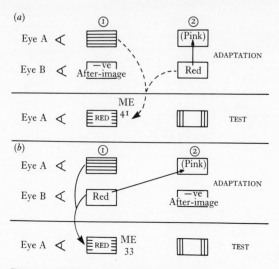

Fig. 15. Dichoptic non-redundant MEs: red induction. (*a*) Pattern alternating with colour; (*b*) pattern simultaneous with colour.

when red was the adapting colour were as follows. When during adaptation eye A saw the horizontal grating and eye B saw the red alternately, a red after-effect, ME strength 41, was set up in association with the horizontal pattern in eye A (fig. 15(*a*)), while the horizontal pattern as seen by eye B was greenish. There was no detectable colouring of the vertical component of the test pattern in either eye. During adaptation it was noticeable that the red not only induced a bluish-green negative after-image in eye B, but also, simultaneous with its presentation, a strongly pink positive after-image in eye A. This positive after-image seen by the pattern-stimulated eye alternately with the pattern is probably responsible for the McCollough effect seen by the pattern-stimulated eye. The mechanism may be as follows. The positive after-image (reddish) set up in eye A during the inter-pattern intervals of adaptation is itself able to produce the equivalent of a negative after-image (greenish) in this eye while the pattern is being viewed, and in consequence it sees a red after-effect on test.

It is remarkable that when a McCollough effect is produced by a pattern alternating dichoptically with a colour, the part of the test pattern corresponding to the adapting pattern is associated with a phantom red, whether the adapting colour is red (fig. 15(*a*)) or green (fig. 14(*a*)). Alternate green may produce its effect through the reddish negative after-image in eye B causing a weak reddish after-image to be set up in eye A during the inter-pattern interval, which then produces the equivalent of a very weak greenish after-image superimposed on the pattern. This roundabout route might account for the extreme weakness of the ME produced by alternate green, compared with that produced by alternate red.

When eye A and eye B were presented with the adapting horizontal grating and red respectively at the same time, eye A on test saw a red McCollough effect of strength ME = 33 associated with the horizontal pattern, while eye B saw a green McCollough effect associated with the vertical pattern (fig. 15(*b*)). Again the red adapting colour induced not only a negative after-image in eye B, but also in pink positive after-image in eye A. It appeared weaker than the positive after-image of the previous experiment (fig. 15(*a*)), presumably because it was not being set up simultaneously with the presentation of the red adapting colour, and this may account for the relative weakness of the ME when pattern and red have been presented simultaneously to the two eyes. The presence of the pattern viewed by eye A appears to prevent the appearance of a simultaneous positive after-image in that eye. This pattern produces the effect of the same pattern being seen simultaneously with red in eye B, hence the relatively strong green McCollough effect seen by eye B in association with the horizontal component of the test pattern.

The results of red induction of non-redundant dichoptic McCollough effects can be summed up as follows. A red after-effect is produced in association with the portion of the test pattern that corresponds to the adapting pattern, whether the adapting colour is presented simultaneously with the adapting pattern or alternately. Pattern and alternate red produce a stronger red McCollough effect than pattern and simultaneous red. On the other hand, pattern and simultaneous red produce a stronger green McCollough effect than pattern and alternate red. Comparing red and green non-redundant dichoptic induction, one can say that in all cases the after-effects are related to the element of the test pattern with the same orientation as the adapting pattern. The strongest red after-effects are formed in the pattern-stimulated eye by pattern and alternate red, and in the colour-stimulated eye by pattern and simultaneous green. A moderately strong red after-effect is formed in the pattern-stimulated eye by pattern and simultaneous red, and a very weak red after-effect is formed, also in the pattern-stimulated eye, by pattern and alternate green. These inter-relationships are crucial to the understanding of redundant dichoptic effects, and especially the so-called 'anomalous' McCollough effect induced in the pattern-stimulated eye as described by MacKay and MacKay (1973, 1975).

Redundant dichoptic effects

In the MacKays' dichoptic experiment (1973, 1975a), eye A sees during adaptation two contrasting patterns presented alternately, and eye B sees two opponent colours, so that each pattern has a simultaneous and an alternate colour with which it can interact. The MacKays reported that the McCollough effect seen by the colour-stimulated eye was normal, in the sense that the pattern that was seen by eye A *at the same time* as a particular colour by eye B, evokes the opponent colour in eye B during testing. On the other hand, the after-effect in the pattern-stimulated eye was held to be anomalous, in that the colour seen on testing in association with a particular pattern was the same as that which coincided in time with that pattern during adaptation. I have repeated the MacKay experiment with the following results. During adaptation eye A saw a horizontal grating while eye B was seeing red, and a vertical grating while eye B was seeing green. On testing, eye B saw a green McCollough effect associated with the horizontal grating, and a red McCollough effect associated with the vertical grating, just as in the MacKays' account. The strength of the red component was ME = 35. Eye A saw a red McCollough effect associated with the horizontal grating, also with a strength of ME = 35, but the vertical grating was colourless (fig. 16). These findings are explicable in terms of the various non-redundant influences present.

It is clear from the analysis that has been made of non-redundant dichoptic effects that the apparent dissociation between the McCollough effects set up in eyes A and B is due mainly to the effects of pattern plus simultaneous red and of pattern plus simultaneous green (fig. 16). The former produces the red after-effect associated with the horizontal grating in eye A, and the green after-effect associated with this pattern in eye B; the latter produces

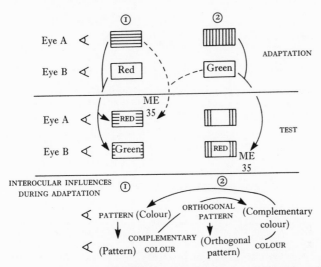

Fig. 16. Dichoptic redundant MEs (MacKay and MacKay, 1973, 1975*a*). Interocular influences: pattern + simultaneous green; pattern + simultaneous red; (pattern + alternate green). Effect of pattern + alternate red cancelled by effect of pattern + simultaneous green.

the red after-effect associated with the vertical grating in eye B. The red after-effect in eye A will be augmented by the weak effect of pattern plus alternate green, and so comes to have a strength equal to that produced in eye B by pattern plus simultaneous green, which is otherwise a more powerful influence than pattern plus simultaneous red. Pattern plus simultaneous green would normally set up a greenish after-effect associated with the vertical pattern in eye A, but this is offset by the red after-effect due to pattern plus alternate red. In consequence the vertical grating in the test pattern is seen as colourless by eye A. The interocular influences that may be at work during adaptation are indicated in fig. 16.

An interesting comparison can be made between the MacKay experiment and a semi-dichoptic experiment described by Dr Keith White in an address given by him to a meeting of the Craik Club in Cambridge University Department of Physiology in 1977. In White's experiment, the pattern-stimulated eye was also colour-stimulated; in other words, this eye (eye A in fig. 17(*b*)) is used to set up an ordinary redundant monocular McCollough effect. The other eye (eye B) is presented with an alternation of colours in phase

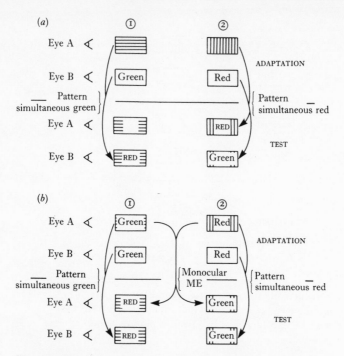

Fig. 17. Dichoptic redundant MEs. (*a*) Orthogonal patterns, complementary colours (see also fig. 16). (*b*) Eye B colour stimulated, eye A pattern and colour stimulated (White's experiment).
Pattern + simultaneous colour mechanisms give the effect of interocular transfer of the monocular ME.

with those seen by eye A, and those colours, in conjunction with the patterns seen simultaneously by eye A, set up a normal McCollough effect in eye B as in the MacKay experiment (fig. 17(*a*)). In this way, pattern plus simultaneous colour mechanisms give the effect of interocular transfer of the monocular ME from eye A to eye B. When the adaptation colour sequence seen by eye B is reversed, so that red is seen by eye B when eye A sees green and vice versa, no McCollough effect is set up in eye B.

Interocular transfer

Most workers are agreed that there is little or no interocular transfer of a monocularly induced McCollough effect. Mikaelian (1974), on the other hand, has reported a curious type of after-effect in the unadapted eye occurring after prolonged binocular viewing of the test pattern. After several minutes a McCollough effect develops in the unadapted eye which is the reverse of that in the adapted eye, that is to say, green replaces red, and red green. Mickaelian regards this as a 'second order McCollough effect' induced in the unadapted eye by the McCollough colours seen binocularly in the test pattern. However, he quotes Helmholtz in support of the notion that the colours seen by the unadapted eye and so generating the McCollough effect in that eye may be complementaries of the colours seen by the adapted eye. If this is so, the colours seen by the unadapted eye will be similar to the colours previously presented to the adapted eye, so that the McCollough effects seen in the two eyes should be the same, not reversed.

I have tried unsuccessfully to replicate Mikaelian's results using my own equipment. A typical experiment was as follows. The adapting gratings were viewed monocularly for the usual 5 minutes, the other eye being kept closed. The unadapted eye was then tested, and no transfer was found to have occurred. The test pattern was then viewed binocularly for 5 minutes. At the beginning of this period the strength of the McCollough effect seen by the adapted eye was ME = 50; at the end of the period it had fallen to ME = 41. The test pattern was then viewed by the unadapted eye only. A McCollough effect was now present; it was not reversed, and its strength was the same as in the adapted eye. In general, I have found that if one eye is kept closed during adaptation no McCollough effect transfers to that eye *until the adapted eye has been tested*. Once a McCollough effect has been seen by the adapted eye, however, a weak but measurable after-effect appears in the unadapted eye. Fig. 18(*a*) illustrates one of many experiments showing this. The dominant eye was adapted. The non-dominant eye was tested, and the ME strength was 0. The dominant eye was found to have an ME of 50. The non-dominant eye was retested immediately; green and red after-effects were present, and the ME strength was 32. Similar results are obtained when the non-dominant eye is adapted. In view of the potentiating action that I have found to be exerted by hyoscine on the McCollough effect, I have also looked for a possible influence of this drug on interocular transfer. Fig. 18(*b*) illustrates that the strength of the McCollough effect is enhanced in the non-adapted eye both before and after it has been seen by the adapted eye.

Interocular transfer is much greater if the unadapted eye is kept

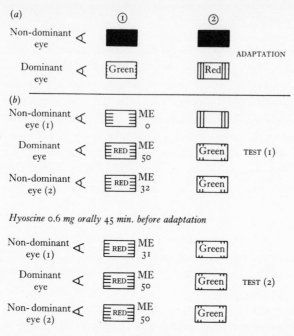

Fig. 18. Monocular redundant MEs: one eye closed. Initial absence of interocular transfer. Partial transfer after ME has been seen by stimulated eye. Interocular transfer enhanced by hyoscine.

open during adaptation and is exposed to white light. A typical such experiment is illustrated in fig. 19. The dominant eye was adapted. The non-dominant eye was tested immediately after adaptation, and was found to have a weak but measurable McCollough effect of ME = 27. The dominant eye had a McCollough effect of ME = 50. The non-dominant eye on retest had an ME of 50, i.e. the same as in the dominant eye, and the same value was obtained when both eyes were tested together. Comparing the results obtained with both eyes open and with one eye closed, we see that with the non-adapted eye open some transfer occurs initially, and is complete when the adapted eye has been tested.

The problem remains, why was the after-effect induced in the unadapted eyes of many subjects in Mikaelian's experiment seen as reversed? A possible clue may lie in the different nature of his test stimulus, which consisted of a hand-held glossy photograph of grating patterns (reproducing those used for adaptation) in which the spaces were considerably wider than the bars. The McCollough

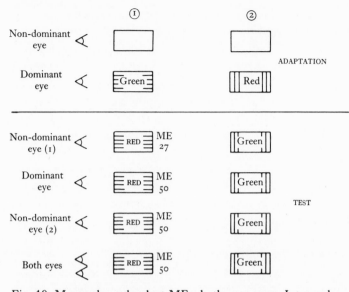

Fig. 19. Monocular redundant MEs: both eyes open. Interocular transfer enhanced.

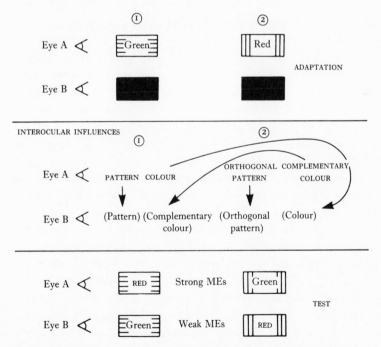

Fig. 20. Monocular redundant MEs. Interocular influences during adaptation tend to set up a weak reversed ME in the unstimulated eye.

effects seen under these conditions were probably much less intense than those produced with slide viewers, and may have less tendency to mask other after-effects set up in the unadapted eye through ocular interaction. My non-redundant dichoptic experiments showed that presentation of an adapting pattern to one eye tends to produce the effect of that pattern simultaneously in the other eye, whereas presentation of an adapting colour to one eye tends to produce the effect of that colour subsequently in the other eye, or of the complementary colour simultaneously, much as described by Helmholtz. The effect of this is to cause a weak reversed McCollough effect to be set up in the non-adapted eye, which under most conditions is masked by partial interocular transfer of the strong McCollough effect set up in the adapted eye (fig. 20).

McCollough effects in amblyopia

The interocular influences that occur during monocular induction of the McCollough effect are not merely of academic interest, since there are important implications relating to amblyopia – the condition where there is impaired vision in one eye, which when associated with a past history of squint is commonly known as 'lazy eye'. I have studied the McCollough effect in a number of amblyopic students picked out on the basis of their inability to perceive stereopsis. None could see the depth illusion when presented with random dot stereograms, and all gave a childhood history of squint. Each subject was asked first to describe the test pattern as seen by the amblyopic eye so that an idea could be obtained of the severity of the condition. A McCollough effect was then induced binocularly in the usual way, and was measured first in the amblyopic eye, then in the normal eye, then again in the amblyopic eye, and finally once more in the normal eye. In most amblyopes, and especially in those with a severe degree of visual impairment so that the adapting pattern was not clearly seen by the defective eye, the McCollough effect when first tested in the impaired eye was weak or absent. After a McCollough effect had been seen by the good eye, the amblyopic eye always registered a measurable McCollough effect, indicating that the interocular transfer which occurs in normal subjects had not been interfered with. In a number of subjects the strength of the after-effect in the amblyopic eye once transfer had occurred was greater than it had

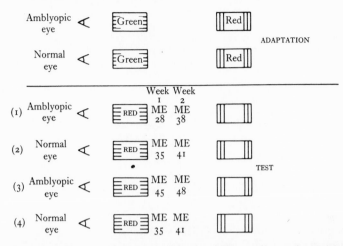

Fig. 21. ME in amblyopia (strabismic). ME usually weaker initially in amblyopic eye, may be stronger in amblyopic eye than in normal eye after transfer.

been in the normal eye, and remained so when that eye was retested. This finding was particularly striking in the experiment illustrated in fig. 21 (see also Campbell *et al.*, 1978*a*), where the subject's amblyopia was so severe that she could not distinguish the direction of the bars in the test pattern. In spite of this, when tested she saw McCollough colours in the appropriate areas of the pattern.

The exceptionally strong McCollough effect seen in the amblyopic eye of a fatigued subject has already been mentioned (chapter 4). Since there is reason to believe that the McCollough effect is primarily an inhibitory phenomenon, the present results raise the question of whether there is an inhibitory factor contributing to the visual impairment in amblyopia. The high McCollough strengths could then be explained as an inhibition superimposed in inhibition. As many have thought, the lazy eye of amblyopia may well have features in common with the ocular dominance produced in cats when one eye has been kept temporarily closed during a critical period of post-natal development (Hubel and Wiesel, 1970; Blakemore and van Sluyters, 1974). There is evidence that the visual defect due to monocular deprivation is caused by influences from the normal eye setting up an inhibitory state in the deprived eye, since the effects are reversed by removal of the normal eye (Kratz

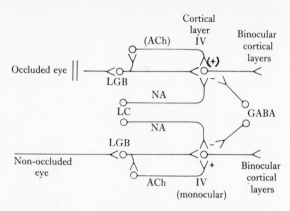

Fig. 22. Increased inhibition due to eye occlusion. Abbreviations: ACh acetylcholine; NA noradrenaline; GABA γ-aminobutyric acid; LGB lateral geniculate body; LC locus ceruleus.

et al., 1976) and by the administration of bicuculline, which blocks the receptors for the inhibitory neurotransmitter γ-aminobutyric acid (GABA), as shown by Duffy *et al.*, (1976). Furthermore, monocularly deprived kittens are protected from ocular dominance by the non-deprived eye by intraventricular injection or local perfusion of 6-hydroxydopamine (6-OHDA) which depletes the brain of catecholamines, and the protection afforded by 6-OHDA is reversed by local perfusion of noradrenaline (Kasamatsu and Pettigrew, 1976; Pettigrew and Kasamatsu, 1978). The significance of these findings probably lies in the fact that in most regions of the brain, including cerebral cortex (Krnjević and Phillis, 1963*a*, *b*, *c*), noradrenaline has an inhibitory effect on cell firing. Suppression of input from the deprived eye through collaterals to the cholinergic reticular activating system may lead to a modulatory imbalance due to relative over-activity of the inhibitory systems (fig. 22).

If there is indeed an inhibitory element in amblyopia, there must be hope that the condition can be ameliorated by procedures designed to break the inhibition. Remarkable improvement has been obtained recently in amblyopic children by causing them to watch revolving achromatic gratings with the amblyopic eye (Campbell *et al.*, 1978*b*). The results of this treatment can be compared with the extinction of the McCollough effect achieved by the repeated presentation of orthogonal achromatic gratings (Skowbo *et al.*, 1974; see fig. 4). The changing orientations of gratings possibly have the effect of stimulating the cholinergic system and so countering inhibitory influences. Since alternating colours when combined with an orthogonal grating pattern have also been found to be highly efficient in expunging the McCollough effect (see chapter 3), it would be interesting to discover whether they could augment the effects of revolving gratings and so prove helpful in amblyopia.

Interocular transfer – addendum
White *et al.* (1978, *Vision Res.* **18**, 1201–15) have recently shown that a monocularly induced McCollough effect is transferred to the contralateral eye when that eye is subjected during adaptation to the same alternation of colours as the adapting eye. Their findings and mine both suggest that opaque occlusion leading to dark adaptation of the non-adapting eye may have a positively suppressive (inhibitory) effect on such interocular transfer as might otherwise occur.

6

DECAY OF THE McCOLLOUGH EFFECT

Pure match and pure null measuring methods

Perhaps the most significant thing to come out of the present studies is the finding that for any subject, the rate of decay of the McCollough effect is determined in a predictable way by the initial strength. Once the first reading has been taken, so long as regular tests are made, the subsequent course of the decay can be foreseen, and any deviation therefore from the expected course that may result from external influences or other factors can be at once determined. It is only necessary that the subject should have been tested previously to establish the value of a '*decay constant*', which varies between individuals, but in any particular subject does not change. The pattern of decay is not peculiar to the match interference method: it seems that any measuring method that is sufficiently sensitive will give similar results, so long as it is based on a simple match or a simple cancellation of the phantom colour or colours. The more complex measuring method of the MacKays leads to a different type of decay, which is analysed in section 2 of this chapter.

Fig. 23 shows two decay curves obtained in myself from measurements made every 12 minutes over a period of 2 hours. One had an initial strength of $ME_0 = 60$, and the other an initial strength of $ME_0 = 48$. The low initial strength was obtained by viewing the adapting slide for the usual 5 minutes through two pieces of Polaroid with their transmission axes set at $45°$. According to the formula given in chapter 4 for the effects of reduced luminance ($ME = \frac{7}{15}ME_0\,I^{1/6}$; see fig. 8), the initial strength

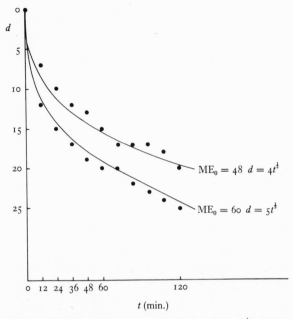

Fig. 23. Normal decay curves given by $d = at^{1/3}$, where d = decrement below initial strength, t = time in minutes, a = initial strength (ME_0) × decay constant ($\frac{1}{12}$ for this subject).

without polars would have been $\text{ME}_0 = 61$. Both curves have a parabola-like appearance, or, more strictly, that of a hemiparabola using the term in its looser sense to indicate a power function not necessarily a quadratic. It is clear from their shapes that the curves take their origin from the points representing the readings for the initial strength. For this reason, if the curves are to be analysed by plotting them with logarithmic co-ordinates, it is essential that the ME strengths should be expressed, not directly in the conventional manner, but as decrements below the initial strength.

Double logarithmic plots of decrement d against time in minutes t for the two curves are shown in fig. 24. In each case the plots are linear with a gradient of $1/3$. In the case where $\text{ME}_0 = 60$, the intercept on the ordinate is 5, giving the equation of the curve as

$$d = 5t^{1/3}$$

Since $d = \text{ME}_0 - \text{ME}_t$ and $5 = \frac{1}{12}\text{ME}_0$, the equation can be written

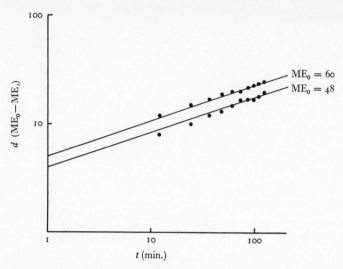

Fig. 24. ME decay curves with different initial strengths in subject with decay constant $\frac{1}{12}$. Log–log plots of decrements ($d = \mathrm{ME}_0 - \mathrm{ME}_t$) against time.

$$1 - \frac{\mathrm{ME}_t}{\mathrm{ME}_0} = \tfrac{1}{12} t^{1/3}$$

In the case where $\mathrm{ME}_0 = 48$, the intercept is 4, giving the equation as

$$d = 4 t^{1/3}$$

Since $4 = \frac{1}{12}\mathrm{ME}_0$ for this curve, the equation is again

$$1 - \frac{\mathrm{ME}_t}{\mathrm{ME}_0} = \tfrac{1}{12} t^{1/3}$$

It should be pointed out that this analysis of the logarithmic plots is based on many experiments, and not just these two curves. The term $1 - (\mathrm{ME}_t/\mathrm{ME}_0)$ will be referred to as the *fractional decrement*. $\frac{1}{12}$ is my decay constant.

The time exponent of 1/3 in the above equations is invariable. The decay constant, as already stated, varies between individuals, although $\frac{1}{12}$ is a rather common value. My research student Mr Amure has a decay constant of $\frac{1}{9}$, which means that he has a natural decay rate which is faster than mine (fig. 25). Log–log plots of the *percentage decrement* $= 100[1 - (\mathrm{ME}_t/\mathrm{ME}_0)]$ against time for

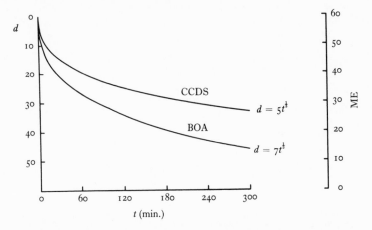

Fig. 25. ME decay curves for subjects with different decay constants (CCDS $\frac{1}{12}$; BOA $\frac{1}{9}$).

subjects with decay constants of $\frac{1}{12}$ and $\frac{1}{9}$ are shown in fig. 31. For a subject regularly testing with a decay constant of $\frac{1}{12}$, the ME will be totally expunged after $(12)^3$ minutes, i.e. after about 29 hours, and for a subject with a decay constant of $\frac{1}{9}$, after $(9)^3$ minutes, i.e. 12 hours. Needless to say, tests are not in practice carried out this long. Also, an ME strength of less than 23 is not measurable.

I have emphasised that decay curves of normal shape occur only if the subject is regularly tested. The precise frequency of the tests is not crucial: for instance, I have obtained an absolutely normal decay curve testing every 36 minutes, that is, three times less frequently than usual. There is no doubt, however, that very infrequent testing leads to slowing of decay, and that very frequent or continuous testing accelerates it. It is probable that little decay occurs before the first test, as Holding and Jones (1976) have pointed out, so there is no need to hurry to do the first test after adapting. Fig. 26 illustrates an experiment in which one eye received its first test 36 minutes after the other, and during that period a decrement of 8 occurred in the eye with delayed testing, as compared with the decrement of 15 in the eye that was tested immediately. It is of course, possible that less decay occurs when testing is delayed in both eyes so that no interocular influences can occur. However, during a period when I was habitually obtaining an initial strength of $ME_0 = 60$ after binocular adaptation, when

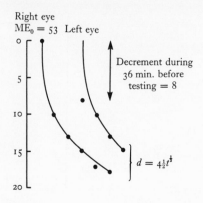

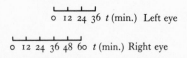

Fig. 26. ME decay rate with delayed testing. One eye received first test 36 minutes after other eye. Decrement during this period = 8.

the first test was delayed 1 hour the initial reading was ME = 50 instead of the expected ME = 40 when there is normal decay. In both these cases, therefore, the decrement was reduced by about $\frac{1}{2}$ by delaying testing.

The normal curves published by Skowbo *et al.* (1974) and derived from matching measurements were averaged from several subjects, but they are very close to those obtained from a subject with a decay constant of $\frac{1}{12}$ (fig. 4). White (1977) has a 200 minute decay curve for which he himself was the subject, constructed from measurements made by the null method of Riggs *et al.* (1974). Only a small depression of the second half of the curve is required to turn it into a power function, and the curve so modified appears to be at least as good a fit for the actual readings as the one which White has drawn. I have made a log–log plot of decrements against time for this modified curve, taking the initial strength W_0 to be 5.7 in White's units (fig. 27). The gradient is 1/3 and the intercept on the ordinate is 0.63, so the equation can be written

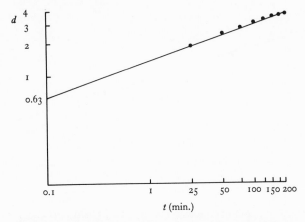

Fig. 27. Null method of Riggs *et al.* (1974). Log–log plot of decrements against time: data from White (1977). Evidence that decay constant for this subject is ⅑ (see text).

$$d = 0.63t^{1/3}$$
$$= \tfrac{1}{9}W_0 t^{1/3}$$

One may conclude that White's decay constant is ⅑ (the same as that of Amure). The fractional decrement for this curve is equal to $\tfrac{1}{9}t^{1/3}$, and the percentage decrement is given by

$$100\left(1 - \frac{W_t}{W_0}\right) = 11t^{1/3}$$

The percentage decrement is plotted against time in fig. 31, where it may be compared with a similar plot for a subject with a decay constant of $\tfrac{1}{12}$.

The MacKay null plus match method

The extraordinarily rapid early decay obtained by the MacKays, quite different from anything got by other measuring methods, can only be clearly seen in decay curves plotted with linear co-ordinates (see MacKay and MacKay, 1977). Mostly the MacKays present their results in logarithmic plots of McCollough effect strength (not decrements), as measured in their arbitrary units, against time. Such plots are approximately linear, with a gradient originally stated to be 1/3 (MacKay and MacKay, 1974) but later given as

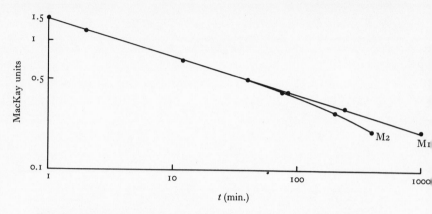

Fig. 28. Null match method of MacKay and MacKay (1973, 1975*a*).
Linear log–log plot of arbitrary units of strength against time (M1: data
from MacKay and MacKay, 1975*a*). For basis of modified plot M2, see
text.

3/10 (MacKay and MacKay, 1975*a*, *b*). The rate of decay appears
to be comparable to that of the decay phase of positive after-images
produced by white light (Padgham, 1965).

In an attempt to relate the MacKay decay curves to those
obtained by other workers, I chose to analyse one of their logarithmic plots (MacKay and MacKay, 1975*a*) in which the adaptation
time was 5 minutes – the same as that used by myself (the MacKays
often use longer adaptation times). The hope was that similar
adaptation times would have led to roughly similar initial strengths,
thereby facilitating comparison of the two curves. On this basis, the
initial strength when measured in MacKay units is $\frac{1}{40}$th of what it
is when measured in my (ME) units which, it will be remembered,
represent the percentage suppression of green light required to
produce the McCollough red. I found that there was not a
consistent relationship between the MacKay curve as published
and my decay curve at corresponding time intervals, if the MacKay
curve was truly linear throughout its length on a log–log plot. If,
however, its course was depressed somewhat after 40 minutes,
then values could be obtained for the MacKay strength which
when plotted against the equivalent ME values gave a smooth curve
(Shute, 1977*c*). The minimum detectable strength (0.2 units by
the MacKay method, ME = 23 by my method) occurred after 400

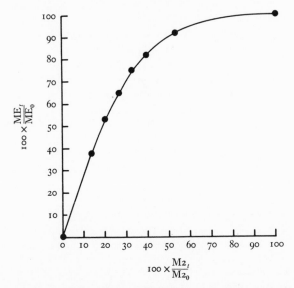

Fig. 29. ME and MacKay (M2) decay curves: equivalent percentages of initial strengths.

minutes in each case, so that this point lay on the curve, as did zero strength.

I have called the modified MacKay curve M2, to distinguish it from M1 which is linear on a log–log plot (fig. 28). M2 begins to diverge from M1 after 40 minutes. The minimum detectable value occurs after 400 minutes on M3 but after 1000 minutes on M1. Some of the MacKays' records do in fact show a number of later readings lying below M1, though not always as low as M2. It is possible that the relatively fewer readings that appear to have been taken in the later stages of some of the experiments may have led to higher values of the McCollough strength.

Fig. 29 shows a comparison between the ME and M2 curves when equivalent strengths are plotted as a percentage of the initial strength in each case, i.e. $100 \times ME_t/ME_0$ is plotted against $100 \times M2_t/M2_0$, where ME_t, $M2_t$ are equivalent strengths after times t, and ME_0, $M2_0$ are the initial strengths in each case. It will be seen that the curve has the shape of a hemiparabola with its origin at the point representing the initial strengths. This suggested that a log–log plot of the percentage decrements would be linear, which proved to be the case. Fig. 30 shows such a plot of

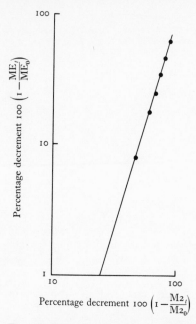

Fig. 30. Relationship between ME and MacKay (M2) decay curves: log–log plot of equivalent percentage decrements.

$100[1-(ME_t/ME_0)]$ against $100[1-(M2_t/M2_0)]$, giving a straight line with a gradient of 10/3, and an intercept on the abscissa of 25. From this we can write the equation

$$25\left[100\left(1-\frac{ME_t}{ME_0}\right)\right]^{0.3} = 100\left(1-\frac{M2_t}{M2_0}\right),$$

whence

$$\left(1-\frac{ME_t}{ME_0}\right)^{0.3} = 1-\frac{M2_t}{M2_0}$$

The above equation gives the relationship between the M2 curve and the McCollough decay curves obtained by simple match and null methods. Fig. 31 shows a log–log plot of the M2 percentage decrement against time for comparison with similar plots for the White and Shute decay curves. The gradients of the latter two curves are both 1/3, and intercepts on the ordinate are respectively 11 and 8, so that the percentage decrements are $11t^{1/3}$ and $8t^{1/3}$,

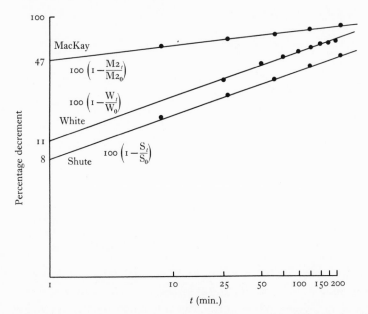

Fig. 31. Comparison of decay curves (MacKay, White, Shute): Log–log plots of percentage decrements against time.

and the fractional decrements are $\frac{1}{9}t^{1/3}$ and $\frac{1}{12}t^{1/3}$ respectively. In the case of the M2 plot, the gradient is $1/10$ and the intercept on the ordinate is 47. The percentage decrement, therefore, is given by

$$100\left(1 - \frac{M2_t}{M2_0}\right) = 47t^{1/10}$$

and the fractional decrement by

$$1 - \frac{M2_t}{M2_0} = \tfrac{8}{17}t^{1/10}$$

Validity of the decay equation

We have seen that, for a subject with a decay factor of $\frac{1}{12}$, during the period that is testable or is normally tested the decay of the McCollough effect is accurately characterised by the equation

$$\left.\begin{aligned}\frac{ME_t}{ME_0} &= 1 - \tfrac{1}{12}t^{1/3} \\[1mm] \text{or}\quad d &= \tfrac{1}{12}ME_0\,t^{1/3}\end{aligned}\right\} \tag{1}$$

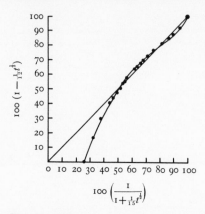

Fig. 32. ME decay rate: alternative equations. Relationship between $1 - \frac{1}{12}t^{1/3}$ and $1/(1 + \frac{1}{15}t^{1/2})$ for different values of t.

One may now ask whether this is 'true' equation, that is, would it continue to describe the decay process equally well if repeated tests were carried out until the McCollough effect was no longer detectable, and beyond that point until the after-effect was completely expunged? Because the graph of a particular equation gives a close approximation to the values obtained during the first few hours of decay, it does not follow that there is no other equation that would also give an adequate match for this period, and might represent more accurately what occurs during the later unmeasured or unmeasurable stages. Consider for instance the equation

$$\left.\begin{array}{c} \dfrac{\text{ME}_t}{\text{ME}_0} = \dfrac{1}{1 + \frac{1}{15}t^{1/2}} \\[1.5em] \text{or its equivalent} \\[1em] d = \dfrac{\text{ME}_0\, t^{1/2}}{15 + t^{1/2}} \end{array}\right\} \qquad (2)$$

Fig. 32 shows a linear plot of $100(1 - \frac{1}{12}t^{1/3})$ against $100/(1 + \frac{1}{15}t^{1/2})$. The graph makes it clear that from zero time to about 6 hours the two expressions are very close, and it is easily shown that this is because, over the time range, $12t^{1/2}/t^{1/3}$ is approximately equal to $15 + t^{1/2}$, and almost exactly so when $t = 15$ or 180.

The closeness of the two expressions for ME_t/ME_0 during the

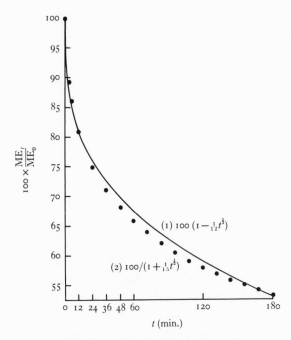

Fig. 33. ME decay rate: alternative equations

(1) $\dfrac{ME_t}{ME_0} = 1 - \frac{1}{12}t^{1/3}$ (solid line)

(2) $\dfrac{ME_t}{ME_0} = \dfrac{1}{1 + \frac{1}{15}t^{1/2}}$

period in which it is possible to measure it can be seen by comparing the two values for the 'half-life': 216 minutes according to equation (1) and 225 minutes according to equation (2). After a lapse of 6 hours the expressions begin to diverge widely, so that after $28\frac{3}{4}$ hours $ME_t/ME_0 = 0$ according to (1), while according to (2) $ME_t/ME_0 = 0.26$ so that when $ME_0 = 60$, $ME_t = 15.6$. This emphasises the most important difference between the two equations, namely that in (1) ME_t/ME_0 reaches zero in finite time, whereas (2) is asymptotic. According to (2), a McCollough effect would never be totally expunged: an initial strength of $ME_0 = 60$ would take just over 2 years to be reduced to 1. The best way to distinguish between (1) and (2) is to conduct a long experiment: the problem being that with an initial strength of 60 the ME reaches the limit of detectability after $6\frac{3}{4}$ hours and becomes difficult to

measure accurately at strengths a bit above this. The longest period
of regular testing that I have carried out has been 5 hours. The value
predicted by equation (1) for ME_t/ME_0 after this period is 0.44,
while that predicted by equation (2) is 0.46. In fact, the value
obtained was 0.44, which favours (1). Fig. 33 shows the forms of
the decay curves given by the two equations over the first 3 hours.
Although the curves are so close, even during this period equation
(1) is the one that usually gives the best fit (see, for example,
fig. 41).

7

EFFECTS OF DRUGS

Methodology

In most of the experiments described in this chapter, the subject, usually myself, adapted for the customary 5 minutes, made the first test to determine the initial strength of the McCollough effect, then took the drug under investigation by mouth. With a few exceptions, the amount taken was the minimum effective clinical dose. Subsequent tests were made at the usual 12-minute intervals for a period of two hours. In most instances the first two or three readings had the values predicted by the normal decay equation, which in my case, since my decay constant is $\frac{1}{12}$, is $d = \frac{1}{12}ME_0\,t^{1/3}$, where d is the decrement below the initial strength ME_0, and t is the time in minutes. Then, as the figures clearly show, a dramatic deviation occurred from the expected course of the decay curve in the case of those drugs which were found to influence the McCollough effect, either downwards to produce lower values and accelerate decay as with coffee or caffeine, or upwards to increase the strength and to slow decay, as with the other drugs. In order to render equivalent the results obtained on different occasions with different initial strengths, the decay curves were recorded by plotting $100 \times ME_t/ME_0$ against t and compared with the normal decay curve given by

$$\frac{ME_t}{ME_0} = 1 - \tfrac{1}{12}t^{1/3}$$

In this way it was possible to make satisfactory comparisons between the effects of different drugs and of different doses of the

Table 13

t (min)	$100(1-\frac{1}{12}t^{1/3})$	t (min)	$100(1-\frac{1}{12}t^{1/3})$
0	100	98	62
3	88	108	$60\frac{1}{2}$
6	85	120	59
12	81	132	58
24	76	144	$56\frac{1}{2}$
36	$72\frac{1}{2}$	156	55
48	70	168	54
60	$67\frac{1}{2}$	180	53
72	$65\frac{1}{2}$	200	51
84	$63\frac{1}{2}$	240	48

same drug. Values of $100(1-\frac{1}{12}t^{1/3})$ for different values of t up to 4 hours are given in table 13.

It is clear that for this method to succeed, the first reading must be accurately made. In practice this did not prove a serious problem, since with experience it was found that a reading could be obtained repeatedly to within $\frac{1}{2}$ a degree of rotation of the wave plate, giving an ME range of ± 2 units or a possible error of about 3 per cent. The effect of such an error on the predicted decay curve is small compared with the deviations produced by drugs, which are easily detected because they occur rapidly as the substance is absorbed from the alimentary tract and crosses the blood–brain barrier. If by any chance a false reading is made, this will become apparent with the second or third readings during the period before the drug reaches the central nervous system, and also, of course, in repeats of the experiment.

There have been no previous accounts of pharmacological influences on the McCollough effect apart from a brief report by myself (Shute, 1978).

Agents affecting cholinergic function

The acetylcholine muscarinic blocking drug hyoscine (scopolamine) is able to increase the strength of the McCollough effect in subjects in whom the effect is normally weak. Fig. 34 shows the effect of 0.6 mg hyoscine (twice the minimum effective clinical dose) given orally 45 minutes before adaptation to four such

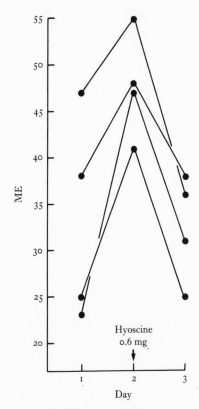

Fig. 34. ME strength. Enhancing effect of 0.6 mg hyoscine given orally 45 minutes before adaptation on second day to four subjects with normally weak MEs.

subjects on the second day in a series of three-day experiments. All the subjects were relatively naive, that is, none had experienced a McCollough effect more than once or twice previously. Apart from the measurements, which speak for themselves, each subject commented on how much more clearly he saw the effect on the second day after taking the drug than on the first or third days when no drug had been taken. Because of these results I was a little surprised to find that when I took the same dose of hyoscine 45 minutes before adaptation the influence of the drug on the strength and decay of my McCollough effect was quite slight. The initial strength was $ME_0 = 60$, which is for me normal. The decay curve was slightly elevated during the first hour, but not by more than

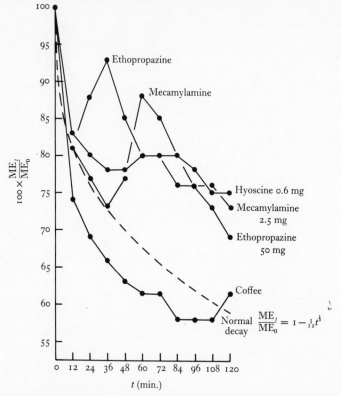

Fig. 35. ME decay rate. Percentage ME plotted against time. Effect of drugs taken orally immediately after first test. Acceleration of decay produced by coffee, deceleration produced by anti-cholinergic drugs. Normal decay given by $ME_t/ME_0 = 1 - \frac{1}{12}t^{1/3}$ (broken line).

3 units. On the other hand, when the hyoscine was taken after adaptation following immediately on the first test, the results were much more impressive (fig. 35). The decay curve began to drop less than the expected amount by the second test, the reading after 1 hour was higher than the two previous ones, and this level was maintained for two more readings before any further decay occurred. In consequence, the ME strength after 84 minutes expressed as a percentage of the initial strength was 80 instead of the expected $63\frac{1}{2}$ (table 13). It appears that hyoscine does not influence the initial strength of a strong McCollough effect, but does arrest decay significantly when given after a McCollough effect has been set up.

Table 14 *Cholinergic agonists* (*a*), *blocking agents* (*b*), *anti-cholinesterases* (*c*, *b*)

(a)

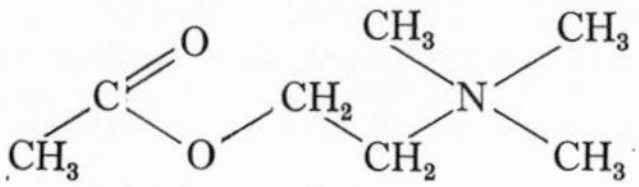

Acetylcholine

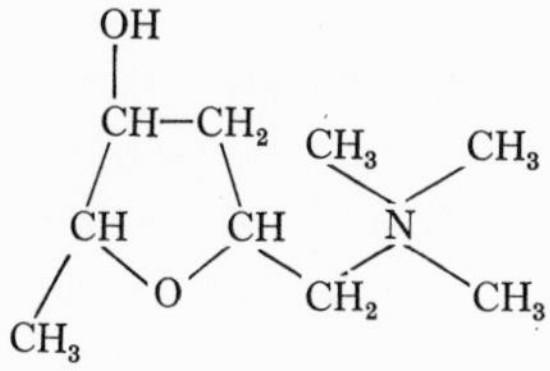

Muscarine

(b)

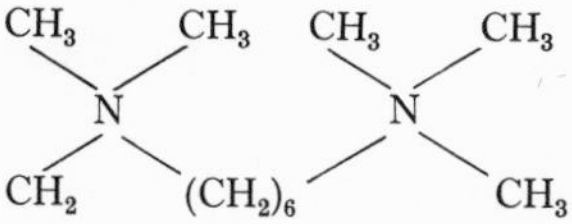

Hexamethonium

PHENOTHIAZINES

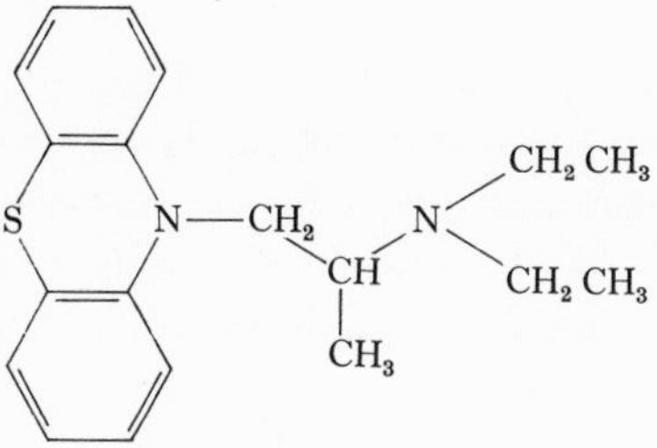

Ethopropazine

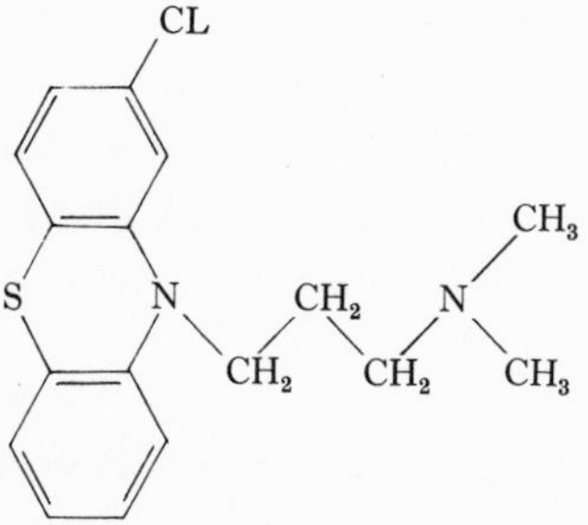

Chlorpromazine

(c)

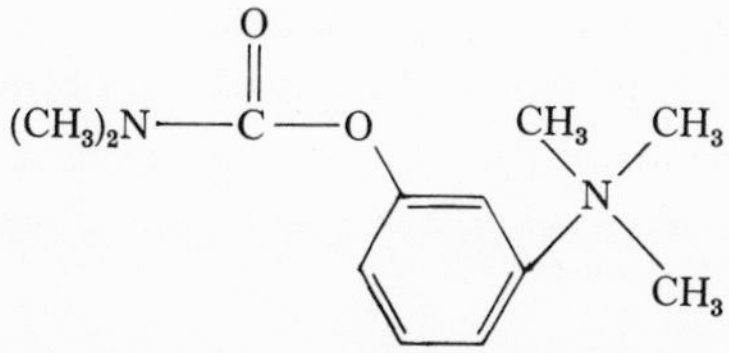

Neostigmine

Because of these findings with hyoscine I tried the effects of two other acetylcholine blocking drugs, ethopropazine – the action of which is similar to that of hyoscine – and the nicotinic blocker mecamylamine, taking in each case the minimum recommended clinical dose immediately after the first test. The resulting decay curves are shown in fig. 35. Ethopropazine is stated to be rather more effective than hyoscine in ameliorating the symptoms of Parkinsonism, where there is an acetylcholine–dopamine imbalance with excessive cholinergic activity due to the loss of the dopamine pathway from the substantia nigra to the corpus striatum. It is interesting, therefore, that ethopropazine caused an early elevation of the McCollough effect strength much greater than that produced by hyoscine, so that after 36 minutes the value of $100 \times ME_t/ME_0$ was 93 instead of the expected $72\frac{1}{2}$.

Ethopropazine is a phenothiazine (table 14) and in its structure is closely related to chlorpromazine, to be discussed later. Like many anti-cholinergic agents, ethopropazine is also an anti-cholinesterase, and indeed is used as such in neurohistochemical procedures: this is because of the structural similarity between cholinesterase and the acetylcholine receptor. However, the effect of the drug in Parkinsonism indicates that the action on cholin-esterase, which would be in the reverse direction, is relatively unimportant clinically, and the response of the McCollough effect bears this out. Mecamylamine is primarily a peripherally active drug, blocking cholinergic transmission in autonomic ganglia. It is known, however, to cross the blood–brain barrier. Its effects when taken by mouth may be slow to appear because of delayed absorption from the gut. Fig. 35 shows clearly that, in the experiment illustrated, decay was normal for the first $\frac{3}{4}$ hour but at 1 hour a peak was reached nearly as great as that produced by ethopropazine.

The results obtained with anti-cholinergic agents can be con-trasted with those produced by coffee or caffeine tablets. Fig. 35 shows that while high ME values and slowed decay are produced by the anti-cholinergic drugs, the effect of coffee is to depress ME levels and accelerate decay during the two-hour period. The curve illustrated was obtained after only one cup containing a teaspoonful of instant coffee. Greater depressions of the McCollough effect are obtained when stronger coffee is taken, such as Cona coffee. These findings suggest that the action of caffeine in the central nervous system is such as to boost cholinergic activity. In fact, two opposed actions have been postulated for caffeine and other xanthines on nervous tissue. On the one hand, it is held that xanthines block the destruction of adenosine-3'-5'-monophosphate (cyclic AMP) by the enzyme phosphodiesterase, so leading to membrane hyperpolarisation and therefore inhibition of cell firing (Greengard *et al.*, 1972). On the other hand, they appear to exert a more direct depolarising influence on the cell membrane and so enhance the excitatory effects of acetylcholine. Furthermore they may increase the release of acetylcholine presynaptically (Matthews and Quilliam, 1964; Crossland, 1971). At present the part played by cyclic AMP in promoting hyperpolarisation appears to be somewhat controversial, and the evidence of the McCollough effect strongly supports a cholinomimetic and cholinagogic role for caffeine. Since acetylcholine is excitatory in the retina (Noell and Lasansky, 1959; Straschill, 1968; Masland and Ames, 1976), at visual relays (Satinsky, 1967) and in the visual cortex (Spehlmann, 1963, 1971), the depression of the McCollough effect produced by caffeine can be regarded as a reversal of inhibition.

Another drug that can have opposing actions on nervous tissue is nicotine. Small doses stimulate acetylcholine receptors in autonomic ganglia and in various medullary and hypothalamic centres, whereas large doses paralyse them. It has been claimed that the psychological consequences of smoking are similarly dosage dependent; according to this view gentle puffing has a stimulatory effect whereas deep inhalation is depressant (Armitage *et al.*, 1968). Amure (1978) has investigated the influences exerted by cigarette smoking and orally ingested nicotine on the McCollough effect. He found no evidence that the initial strength of the after-effect was altered, but the subsequent decay rate was slow in smokers as compared with non-smokers. It was slowed too in subjects who did not normally smoke but were prepared to do so for the purposes of the experiment, and in volunteers taking nicotine by mouth. When considered alongside of the caffeine and hyoscine experiments, these results suggest that nicotine exerts a predominantly sedatory effect, at least as far as the visual system is concerned. One cannot be sure, however, that this sedation is due to a direct depressant action of nicotine on visual centres. Nicotine causes an increased synthesis and release of noradrenaline in the brain (Bhagat, 1970; Hall and Turner, 1972), so that the effects of smoking could be due to stimulation of nicotinic receptors in the locus ceruleus of the hindbrain, which is the source of the main noradrenergic pathways. Since the catecholamine systems of the brain appear to be involved in self-stimulation (Crow, 1972; Phillips and Fibiger, 1973; Lippa *et al.*, 1973), it may be that activation of these systems is responsible for the, to some, pleasurable effects of smoking.

Minor tranquillisers (benzodiazepines)

The benzodiazepines are believed to act by potentiating the central inhibition produced by the inhibitory neurotransmitter γ-aminobutyric acid or GABA (Suria and Costa, 1975; Kozhechkin and Ostrovskaya, 1977). I have investigated the three in most common use, namely diazepam (Valium), chlordiazepoxide (Librium) and nitrazepam (Mogadon). All have essentially similar actions: those of diazepam are illustrated in fig. 36.

The experiments were all performed in the morning at 10 a.m. When 1–2 cups of coffee had been drunk at breakfast 1–2 hours before adaptation, 2.5 mg diazepam taken immediately after the first test had no effect on decay during the first 48 minutes: the decay curve followed exactly its predicted course. There was a very slight elevation of some later readings. When the same dose of diazepam was given without previous coffee, the decay curve began to be elevated at the second reading and the subsequent decay rate was slower than normal. When 5 mg diazepam was taken, the decay curve reached a peak of $100 \times ME_t/ME_0 = 89$ at 36–48 minutes and the subsequent decay was almost parallel to that recorded after half this dose, but at a higher level. Although benzodiazepines are said to take several hours to build up maximal plasma levels, it is clinical experience that effects begin to be felt a few minutes after the drug has been taken. This rapid action is reflected in the shape of the decay curves.

A similar elevation of the decay curve with a peak at 36 minutes occurred when 10 mg chlordiazepoxide was taken without previous coffee (fig. 37). The record obtained when a similar dose of chlordiazepoxide was preceded by coffee showed a depression below the normal curve, presumably due to the coffee, in the first

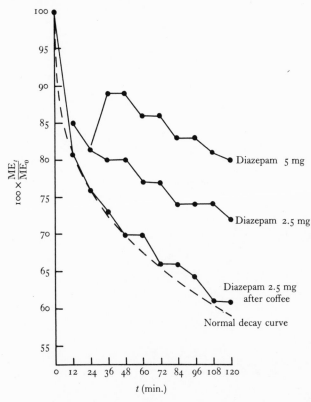

Fig. 36. ME decay rate. Effects of diazepam (Valium), showing dose dependency. Deceleration blocked by coffee taken before adaptation.

hour, and an elevation, presumably due to the drug, during the second hour. The results following 5 mg nitrazepam (fig. 38) were almost identical to those produced by 2.5 mg diazepam. There appears to be little hard evidence for the claim that nitrazepam has a hypnotic action that is different from the tranquillising action of other benzodiazepines.

Some workers have claimed on the basis of animal experiments *in vitro* and *in vivo*, that GABA is not potentiated by benzodiazepines but antagonised by them (Gähwiler, 1976; Steiner and Felix, 1976). According to Gähwiler, working on explants of rat cerebellum, low doses of benzodiazepines act as GABA antagonists whereas high doses act in a GABA-like way and depress cell firing. If these results reflect what occurs when benzodiazepines are

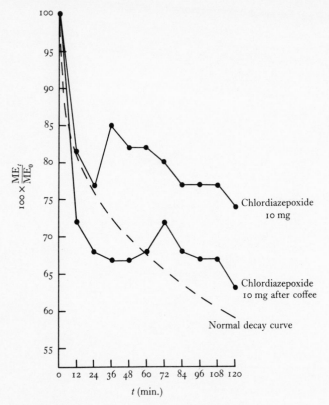

Fig. 37. ME decay rate. Effects of chlordiazepoxide (Librium).

administered to man, one might expect to see a biphasic response in the McCollough decay curve, that is to say, an early depression followed by a later elevation when drug levels have built up. In fact, there is no such early depression: the response is always one of elevation. With high doses the decay process, which can be regarded as a disinhibition, is actually reversed, so that the inhibitory level is increased. The psychophysical measurements, therefore, support the conclusion reached by Kozhechkin and Ostrovskaya (1977) on the basis of recordings from rabbit cerebral cortex, that benzodiazepines act synergically with GABA. The moral seems to be that neuropharmacological findings must sometimes be regarded with caution until fully confirmed, and certainly cannot safely be extrapolated from one central system to another.

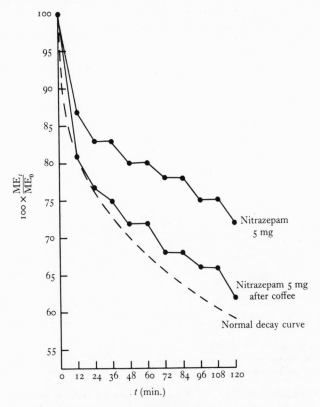

Fig. 38. ME decay rate. Effects of nitrazepam (Mogadon).

Drugs influencing catecholamine systems

In most regions of the brain, including cerebral cortex (Krnjević and Phillis, 1963a, b, c) though not, apparently, the lateral geniculate body (Satinsky, 1967), catecholamines have an inhibitory effect upon cell firing and, therefore, act in opposition to acetylcholine. Consequently, one might expect drugs such as amphetamines that promote the release of catecholamines to elevate the McCollough effect and to slow its decay, and those such as chlorpromazine that block dopamine receptors to act in the reverse direction. As an example of the first class of drugs, I have chosen to study magnesium pemoline (Kethamed) which is safer to use and more suited to experimental use than amphetamine. Pemoline is a phenylethylamine derivative like other sympathomimetic sub-

Table 15 *Sympathomimetic substances (phenylethylamine derivatives)*

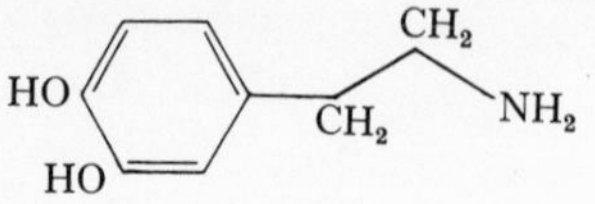

Dopamine

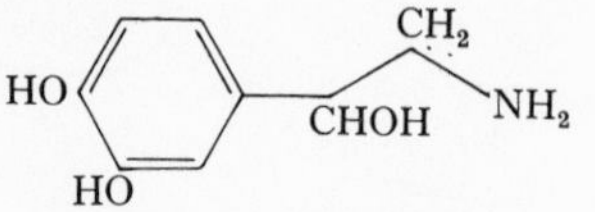

Noradrenaline

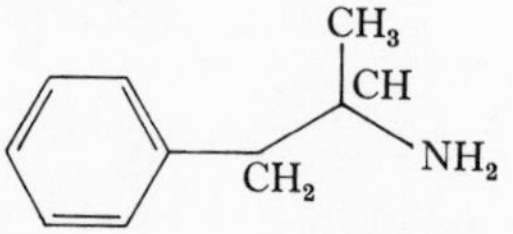

Amphetamine

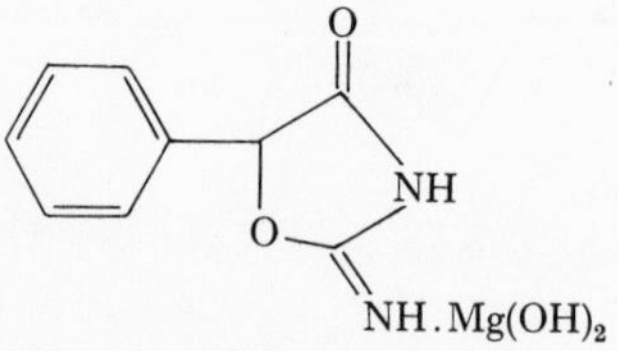

Mg-pemoline

stances, and indeed is a cyclicised compound closely related to amphetamine, as shown by table 15.

Pemoline produces some of the central effects of amphetamine in a mild form, without inducing loss of appetite. Both drugs can induce stereotyped behaviour in the rat (Wallach and Gershon, 1972). Pemoline has been found to stimulate ribonucleic acid synthesis (Glasky and Simon, 1966) and to diminish RNA break-down (Muset *et al.*, 1967) in rats, and also to enhance acquisition and retention of a conditioned avoidance response (Plotnikoff, 1966; Bowman, 1966). Burns *et al.*, (1967) found no enhancement of learning in man with either pemoline or amphetamine, never-theless pemoline has been used in geriatric practice in the treatment of senile amnesia. Success has also been claimed for pemoline as well as for amphetamine as an aid in the management of 'hyper-active' or distractible children (Knights and Viets, 1975).

The action of 40 mg pemoline as reflected in the decay of the McCollough effect is seen in fig. 39. The drug was given, as usual,

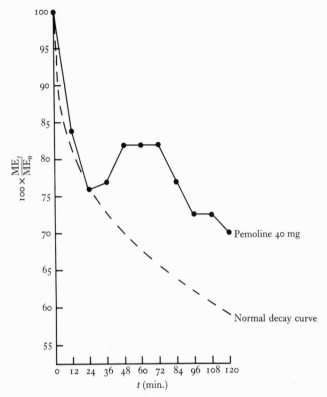

Fig. 39. ME decay rate. Effect of magnesium pemoline.

orally immediately after the first test and reached a plateau during the 48–72 minute period. During this time the value of $100 \times ME_t/ME_0$ was 82, instead of the expected 70 dropping to $65\frac{1}{2}$ (table 13). The role of pemoline in relation to arousal is discussed in chapter 8.

If an amphetamine-like substance that boosts catecholamine activity produces an elevation of the McCollough decay curve, one might expect a drug such as chlorpromazine that blocks dopamine receptors to depress it. Unfortunately information on this point is scanty. A major tranquilliser is not a drug that one cares to use lightly for experimental purposes. Moreover, since chlorpromazine is a phenothiazine, one would expect the initial effect, i.e. that of a single dose, on the decay curve to be like that of ethopropazine, an elevation. Clinical improvement in schizophrenic conditions,

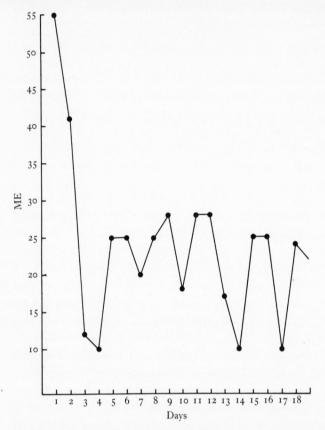

Fig. 40. ME strength in chronic schizophrenic receiving 300 mg/day chlorpromazine. Record started day after clinical exacerbation. Extra 100 mg chlorpromazine given on days 1 and 3.

which is believed to be due to dopamine blockade, does not occur until the drug has been given for some 10 days. I have, however, recorded changes in the strength of the McCollough effect, initial reading only, in a subject diagnosed as a chronic schizophrenic who was receiving a daily maintenance dose of 300 mg chlorpromazine. His normal values were very low, but he was certainly capable of seeing a strong McCollough effect since a fairly high value ($ME_0 = 55$) was recorded during a clinical relapse, which then came down to scarcely measurable levels as the dose of chlorpromazine was increased to 400 mg and his clinical condition improved (fig. 40). There is some evidence that chlorpromazine and other dopamine blockers also promote the synthesis of acetylcholine in the brain (Trabucchi *et al.*, 1974).

Effects of ginseng

The effects of drugs so far recorded seemed to fall into a pattern: one likely to have excitatory effects with respect to cell firing depressed ME strengths and accelerated decay; those likely to have inhibitory effects at the cellular level enhanced the ME strength where that tended to be low, and slowed decay. I thought at this point it would be interesting to test a substance the effects of which could in no way be predicted, and which indeed might well have no effect at all. In other words, the McCollough effect was to be used as a screening procedure for central activity. The substance I had in mind was ginseng.

Ginseng is prepared from the dried root of the plant *Panax ginseng*, so called because it has been regarded as a panacea for a vast range of human ailments including sexual disorders and senility, and as such has been in use in oriental folk medicine for centuries. It has also become something of a cult drug in certain parts of the Western world. The clinical actions most consistently claimed for ginseng have been the production of a state of euphoria and the suppression of fatigue – effects not dissimilar from those produced by amphetamines. Indeed, the euphoria if it occurs could account from some of its alleged therapeutic potency. I have to confess that it was with some scepticism that I tried the effect of 600 mg of a powdered root preparation of Korean ginseng, as supplied by Healthcrafts, Godalming, Surrey, on McCollough decay. I was all the more surprised to find a great elevation of the curve after the second test, reaching a peak at the third test with a value for $100 \times ME_t/ME_0$ of 87 instead of the expected $72\frac{1}{2}$ (fig. 41). On the other hand, a similar test made with Korean instant ginseng tea manufactured by Il Hwa Pharmaceutical Co. Ltd and kindly made available to me from a presentation sample by the President of the Royal Society, Lord Todd, had absolutely no effect on the decay curve, as fig. 41 shows. This result is in accord with other evidence that the freeze-dried instant preparation may be refreshing (to my taste it is definitely not attractive) but lacks therapeutic efficacy (Fulder, 1976).

Ginseng root has been shown to contain a number of substances,

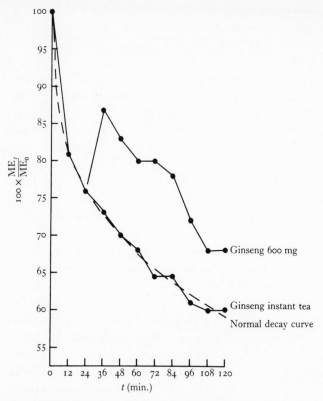

Fig. 41. ME decay rate. Effects of ginseng dried root preparation and ginseng instant tea.

but the active principles are believed to be glycosides, of which the aglycone moiety is a steroid. One such glycoside 20-s-protopanaxadiol with two sugars attached to the steroid skeleton (Fulder, 1977) is shown in table 16, which also indicates some structural affinities not only with adrenocorticosteroids but also with cyclic derivatives of amphetamines acting as monoaminoxidase inhibitors, which may or may not be relevant to their pharmacological effects (information derived from Biel, 1970). Steroids are thought to have some amphetamine-like actions, e.g. the hyperpolarisation of cell membrane due to the activation of cyclic AMP (Robison *et al.*, 1971), so it is possible that ginseng glycosides have similar powers.

Table 16 *Amphetamine derivatives and steroids*

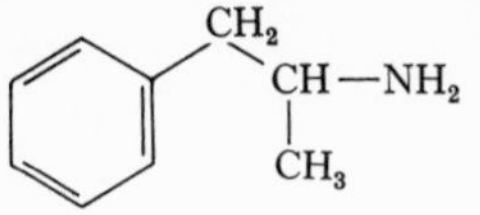

Amphetamine

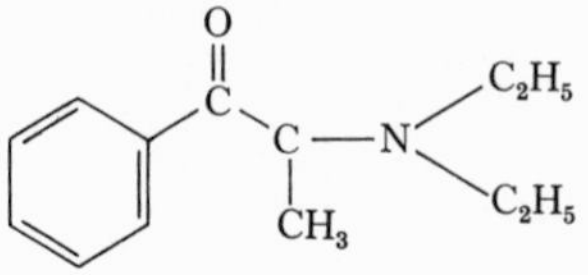

Diethylpropion

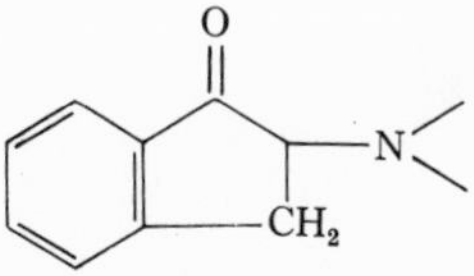

Cyclic derivatives
(= MAO inhibitors)

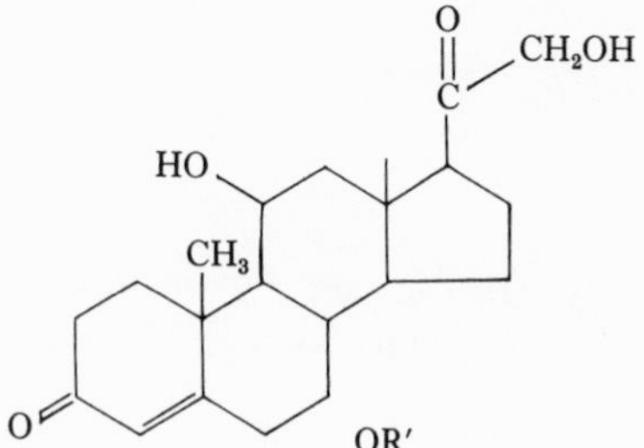

Adrenocorticosteroids

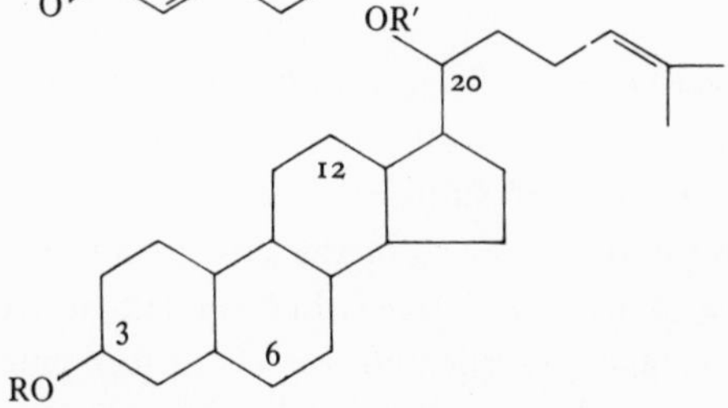

20-s-protopanaxadiol
Ginseng glycoside
(= steroid aglycone +
sugars R,R')

Conclusions

It should not be supposed that all centrally active drugs influence
the McCollough effect. I did not find any change in the decay curve
following 1 mg dihydroergotamine taken sublingually immediately
after the first test. This α-adrenaline blocking agent can cross the
blood–brain barrier and cause toxic central effects, but probably

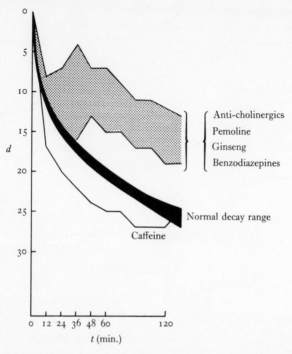

Fig. 42. ME decay rate: influence of drugs. Decrement plotted against time. Acceleration by coffee, deceleration by anti-cholinergic agents, pemoline, ginseng, benzodiazepines.

not in such small dosage. Rather surprisingly, I obtained a normal decay curve during the first $1\frac{1}{2}$ hours after taking 8 ml alcohol (ethanol) in spite of the quite powerful subjective effects produced. The curve did become elevated, however, in the last 30 minutes of the experiment during a 'hang-over' stage when the subjective effects were less pleasant. I have not repeated this procedure, and so am unable to say whether, perhaps, some metabolite of alcohol such as acetaldehyde was on this occasion exerting an influence on decay.

The evidence seems to suggest that the McCollough decay curve may become elevated not through a general depressant of central nervous activity such as alcohol probably is, but through agents which disturb the balance between excitation and inhibition, depressing the former and enhancing the latter. On this hypothesis, increase in the strength of the McCollough effect or a decrease in its decay rate is due to an increased degree of inhibition of the adapting colour channel, brought about by hyperpolarising influences resulting from acetylcholine blockade or from agents that promote catecholamine or GABA activity. A reduction in the strength of the McCollough effect or an increase in its decay rate would be expected to result from depolarising influences, but is much less easily brought about by drugs that are safe to use experimentally. Of substances readily available, only caffeine and related substances seem to be effective: perhaps if other alternatives were obtainable they would become the basis of popular stimulant beverages.

Fig. 42 (Shute, 1978) summarises the effect of drugs on McCollough decay. The ordinate measures decrements below initial strength. The black area gives a range for normal decay rates, since the initial strengths varied. The stippled area lies between the envelopes of the decay curves produced by anti-cholinergic drugs, pemoline, ginseng and minor tranquillisers. The broad base by which the stippled area is connected with the black is due to the slow absorption of mecamylamine. Only the caffeine curve lies below the black. It is suggested that chlorpromazine in dosage sufficient to block dopamine receptors could produce caffeine-like effects: lithium salts through their ability to increase the release of acetylcholine (Paton *et al.*, 1971) might have a similar action.

8

MUSCULAR ACTIVITY, AROUSAL, STRESS

Cholinergic system

If, as the drug experiments described in chapter 7 suggest, decay of the McCollough effect is accelerated and perhaps caused by cholinergic activity, one would expect that measures aimed at increasing this activity such as the application of stress would depress the strength of the after-effect. It is believed, too, that the cholinergic system plays an important part in determining levels of arousal, so that high arousal states could be associated with low McCollough strengths and vice versa. Evidence for cholinergic involvement in arousal is as follows. Electrocortical desynchronisation (high frequency, low amplitude activity), which is an electroencephalographic sign of behavioural arousal, is produced by high-frequency electrical stimulation of the midbrain reticular formation, where many of the nerve cells, particularly the larger ones which are the more readily stimulated, have the histochemical characteristics of cholinergic neurones (Shute and Lewis, 1963, 1967). High frequency stimulation of the midbrain reticular formation also causes acetylcholine to be released from the cerebral cortex (Kanai and Szerb, 1965). Since acetylcholine excites cortical neurones and cortical neurones are known to be hyperactive during desynchronisation, one may conclude that the cholinergic reticular formation plays a fundamental role in arousal, and forms an essential part of the so-called ascending reticular activating system (ARAS). Spehlmann and Downes (1974) and Spehlmann and Smathers (1974) have also provided evidence that acetylcholine acts as an excitatory transmitter in the sensorimotor cortex during the arousal response.

Pavlov (see Gray, 1964) distinguished in his experimental dogs between a 'strong' and 'weak' nervous system, and the Russian school of psychologists, particularly B. M. Taplov and his co-workers, have applied the same distinction to man. A weak nervous system is one that is highly reactive to external stimuli, and a particularly effective marker of this is an excitatory response to caffeine (Rozhdestvenskaya, 1955, reprinted in translation in Gray, 1964). I have suggested (Shute, 1973, 1975) that a weak nervous system may be one in which the cholinergic system is highly active, or it could be that the reactivity of cholinoceptive neurones to the cholinergic input, i.e. the sensitivity of acetylcholine receptors, is more than usually great. The responsiveness to caffeine strongly suggests a cholinergic factor.

A weak nervous system is one which is likely to react strongly to stress, and there is evidence, some of it of a rather indirect nature, that the cholinergic system is involved in the responses of the body to stressful stimuli. First, the ascending sensory pathways of the brain are believed to send collaterals to the (cholinergic) reticular formation. Secondly, the pituitary polypeptides melanocyte-stimulating hormone (MSH) and adrenocorticotrophic hormone (ACTH) are released during stress from the pars intermedia and pars distalis of the adenohypophysis (Sandman *et al.*, 1973; Francis and Peaslee, 1974; Moriarty *et al.*, 1975). MSH and ACTH are similar in chemical constitution and have similar effects on behaviour (Stratton and Kastin, 1973). Since ACTH analogues without corticotrophic activity produce behavioural effects (Bohus *et al.*, 1973; Versteeg, 1973), it is likely that ACTH acts directly on the brain as well as through release of glucocorticoids from the adrenal gland. ACTH was found by Torda and Wolff (1952) to increase the synthesis of acetylcholine in the brain, and increased acetylcholine production is believed to be a concomitant of increased cholinergic activity, e.g. in the retina (Masland and Livingstone, 1976). In Parkinsonism there is a relative excess of cholinergic activity due to the loss of dopamine neurones, and this condition can be aggravated by MSH and relieved by hypothalamic MSH inhibitory factor (Marx, 1975). Glucocorticoids have as their main target cells in the brain the pyramidal neurones of the hippocampus (Gerlach and McEwen, 1972; Rhees *et al.*, 1975). The output from the hippocampus is an excitatory one, and probably facilitates cholinergic activity in the rest of the brain

(a)

(b)

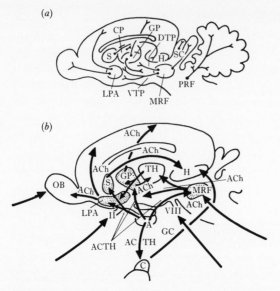

Fig. 43. (*a*) Central cholinergic pathways. Abbreviations: CP caudate and putamen; DTP dorsal tegmental pathway; GP globus pallidus. H hippocampus; LPA lateral preoptic area (substantia innominata); MRF midbrain reticular formation; PRF pontine reticular formation; S septum and diagonal band; SC superior colliculus; VTP ventral tegmental pathway.

(*b*) Stress pathways. Abbreviations: ACh cholinergic neurones; ACTH adrenocorticotrophic hormone; C adrenal cortex; GC adrenal glucocorticoids; MSH melanocyte stimulating hormone; OB olfactory bulb; TH thalamus; II optic nerve; VIII auditory nerve. Other abbreviations as in (*a*). Sites of cholinergic neurones stippled.

(Lewis and Shute, 1967). Hippocampal lesions and anti-cholinergic medication can produce some similar behavioural effects, viz. interference with memory and learning (Bignani and Rosić, 1971) – see chapter 9.

Cholinergic pathways that may be involved in responses to stress are illustrated in fig. 43(*b*). Stress-induced inputs from the olfactory bulb, optic or auditory nerves, and ascending spinal tracts cause ACTH and MSH to be released from the adenohypophysis. These substances act directly or indirectly on cholinergic neurones in the lateral preoptic area (substantia innominata in man), septum, globus pallidus and midbrain reticular formation. Glucocorticoids released from adrenals act on, and may inhibit, the hippocampus.

A thalamic feedback onto cholinergic centres can occur through projections from non-specific thalamic nuclei, e.g. the centro-median nucleus onto the lateral preoptic area and globus pallidus. The arousal responses produced by the dorsal tegmental cholinergic pathway of Shute and Lewis (1963, 1967) are probably elicited by this route.

Measurement of stress

If stress activates the cholinergic system and the McCollough effect is depressed by cholinergic activity, a drop in the strength of the McCollough effect is to be expected when the subject is exposed to a stressful stimulus. In order to investigate this further I have used a device for measuring skin resistance kindly made for me by Mr P. L. Joyce and Mr M. Swann of the Physiological Laboratory, Cambridge. The circuitry is illustrated in fig. 44. A small constant direct current is generated electronically from a battery source and is passed through the skin by surface electrodes which clip onto the thumb and forefinger of one hand. The potential difference between the electrodes is directly proportional to the skin resistance. It is compared with the potential difference produced by a constant backing current passing through a variable resistance ('range' control). Small differences are amplified (the required sensitivity being obtained through a 'gain' control) and displayed on a potentiometer dial. The apparatus was calibrated by putting resistors of known resistance between the electrodes. A convenient setting of the gain control was adopted and then not varied. It was found that 1 unit on the potentiometer scale corresponded to 6 kΩ and 1 unit on the control scale corresponded to 100 kΩ. If the range control reading was R units, and the potentiometer scale reading was V units, values for skin resistance R_s and skin conductance C_s were given by the equations:

$$R_s = 100R - 6V - 224 \text{ k}\Omega$$
$$C_s = \frac{1000}{100R - 6V - 224} \mu\text{mho}$$

Skin conductance can be regarded as a measure of peripheral cholinergic activity. Changes in conductance are believed to be brought about, in the main, by sweating. A rapid transitory increase is known as the galvanic skin reflex and is a component

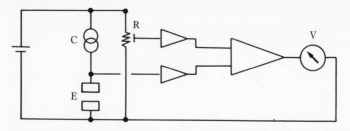

Fig. 44. Skin resistance meter ('stress meter'). For description, see text. Abbreviations: C constant current generator; E skin electrodes; R 'range' control (variable resistance); V potentiometer.

of the 'startle response'. A more sustained increase may occur as a response to stress. As a stressful stimulus I used intense sound produced by an oscillator and delivered to the ears through headphones. Early experiments did show an increase in skin conductance and a small drop in the strength of the McCollough effect, greater than that expected from natural decay, so long as the procedure evoked feelings of anxiety, e.g. relating to possible damage to hearing. Unfortunately, however, with familiarity the stimulation soon ceased to be stressful; little more than a startle response was recorded by the stress meter, and changes in the strength of the McCollough effect were slight or non-existent.

Far more effective than would-be stressful stimuli in causing a decrease in skin resistance were muscular movements. I found that by using the free hand to squeeze vigorously the side of the bench or to manipulate a spring wrist exerciser, the skin resistance could be reduced by 50–100 kΩ in under half a minute. I performed some experiments on myself and other subjects to see whether a reduction in skin resistance produced in this way was accompanied by a decrease in the strength of the McCollough effect. I found that it was. After the initial reading ME_0 had been taken, the squeezing manoeuvre was carried out for 10 seconds and the concomitant decrease in skin resistance was observed. The McCollough effect strength was then remeasured as quickly as possible so as to minimise the amount of natural decay. Making a second reading 15 seconds after an initial reading of $ME_0 = 60$, in a typical experiment I obtained a value $ME_t = 48$ ($t = \frac{1}{4}$ min). This gave a value for the percentage decrement of $100[1 - (ME_t/ME_0)] = 20$, compared with the expected value of $100 \times \frac{1}{12}(\frac{1}{4})^{1/3} = 5\frac{1}{4}$. In other words, the effect of the muscular activity was to increase the percentage decrement by nearly four times. A possible interpretation is that increased peripheral cholinergic activity is accompanied by increased central cholinergic activity, accelerating the decay of the McCollough effect.

I also used the skin resistance meter to compare the effects on arousal of two drugs normally classed as central 'stimulants', namely caffeine and the amphetamine-like substance pemoline. It will be remembered from chapter 7 that these drugs have opposite actions on the McCollough effect: caffeine produces a depression and accelerates decay, whereas pemoline does the reverse. It is indeed a considerable merit of the McCollough effect as a neuro-biological tool that it will readily distinguish between stimulation due to central excitation (caffeine) and stimulation due, presumably, to disinhibition (amphetamines). Both caffeine and pemoline increase the level of arousal as determined by changes in skin resistance. One one occasion the skin resistance dropped from 480 kΩ to 340 kΩ one hour after a cup of coffee; on another occasion it dropped from 660 kΩ to 480 kΩ one hour after 40 mg pemoline. In each case there was a greater decrease than is obtained from muscular activity: typical figures for the squeezing technique are a drop from 660 kΩ to 580 kΩ. Having produced this drop in skin resistance with drugs, I then tried to get a further decrease by squeezing. The results were not the same in the two cases. It was extremely difficult to obtain any further drop in skin resistance after caffeine, but easy after pemoline. It appears that, in Pavlovian terminology, pemoline 'weakens' the central nervous system. These findings may be relevant to the effectiveness of pemoline in the treatment of hyperactive or distractible children (Knights and Viets, 1975). Pemoline may not only increase the general level of arousal, but may also increase the responsiveness to specific arousing stimuli, thereby aiding concentration.

Excessive arousal and transmitter imbalance

There is no reason to suppose that moderate amounts of stress are in any way harmful to the normal individual. Like moderate amounts of muscular exercise, that may have the beneficial effect of toning up the cholinergic system. But there may be dangers in

Table 17

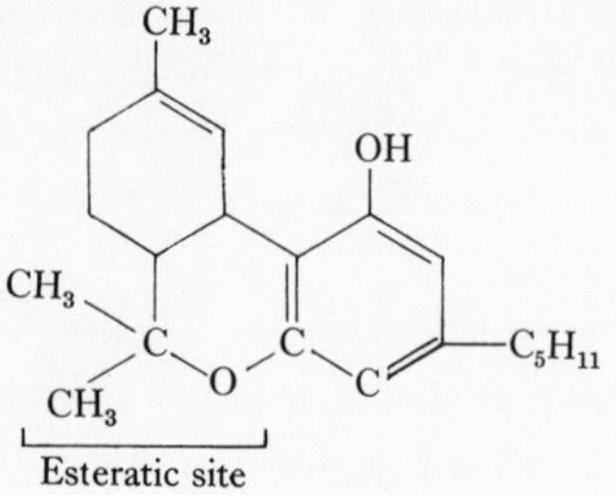

Tetrahydrocannabinol
(THC)

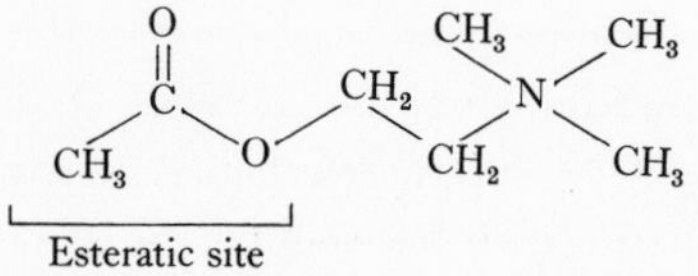

Esteratic site

Acetylcholine

Esteratic site

excess. There is the possibility of positive cholinergic feed-back, since acetylcholine produces release of ACTH-releasing hormone in the hypothalamus (Bradbury *et al.*, 1973; Hillhouse *et al.*, 1975) leading to more cholinergic activity. In susceptible individuals equipped with a 'weak' or hyper-reactive nervous system, or in any individual if circumstances are sufficiently adverse, the over-activity of the cholinergic system induced by prolonged stress is likely to be succeeded by exhaustion phenomena. The synthesis of acetylcholine by the brain is impaired (Torda and Wolff, 1952) and there is diminished release of MSH from the pituitary (Francis and Peaslee, 1974). This is the last stage of Selye's 'general adaptation syndrome'.

The sequence of events outlined above can be severely aggravated by two drugs, either of which can precipitate psychological break-down. First, amphetamine. The effect of amphetamine is to enhance the overactivity and hyper-responsiveness of the cholinergic system. This may precipitate the exhaustion phase. Secondly, cannabis. Many of the effects of cannabis can be attributed to acetylcholine receptor blockade, e.g. dry mouth, rapid pulse, defects in memory, learning and attention. A comparison of the formula of tetrahydrocannabinol (THC), the active principle of cannabis, with that of acetylcholine makes it clear how THC can occupy the esteratic site of the acetylcholine receptor (table 17).

Like other acetylcholine blockers, THC may also show some anti-cholinesterase activity. For an account of the pharmacology of cannabis, see Drew and Miller (1974). The acetylcholine blocking effect may precipitate a neurotransmitter imbalance with a catecholamine excess, particularly excess of dopamine as is believed to occur in schizophrenia.

Since the relative balance of excitatory and inhibitory neurotransmitters is undoubtedly of great importance to the functioning of the individual in health and disease, and since this balance appears to be in part reflected in the behaviour of the McCollough effect, there is an urgent need to learn more about how the McCollough effect varies from person to person and to what extent such variations can be correlated with other individual features. Many questions remain to be answered. Is there, for instance, any relationship between the strength and decay characteristics of the McCollough effect and personality types, degree of introversion or extraversion, etc.? If introversion is characterised by high levels of arousal (see Corcoran and Houston, 1977) and if arousal is positively correlated with cholinergic activity, one might expect the McCollough effects developed by introverts to be relatively weak. Are there characteristics of the McCollough effect that can be related to different types of mental disorder, or to different stages or phases in the disease? I have mentioned in chapter 7 a suspicion that the agitated phase of a schizophrenic attack may be accompanied by relative high McCollough strengths, but this certainly requires confirmation. It is unlikely that psychotics could be persuaded to submit to the tedium of determining decay curves, but the simplicity and portability of the match interference apparatus should make it possible to take initial measurements.

9

LEARNING, MEMORY AND FORGETTING

Effective stimuli

The strongest McCollough effects are achieved when (a) the coloured adapting stimuli consist of two bright, saturated and highly contrasted alternate colour pairs such as red and green which evoke opponent colour responses so that visual neurones that are excited by one colour are inhibited by the other; and when (b) these colours are paired with two strongly contrasting patterns, of which orthogonal gratings are the most effective because their special features, orientated edges with a particular spatial frequency, are ones for which many visual units are coded and specifically respond. Other forms of stimulation, such as movement (Stromeyer and Mansfield, 1970) can be paired with colour to produce a coloured after-effect. If the stimuli paired with colours are contrasting patterns, they must be seen as contrasting patterns and not in some other way if they are to give rise to a McCollough effect. Jenkins and Ross (1977) have made use of a test pattern consisting of a series of concentric squares. This can be seen either as (1) four triangular gratings separated by phantom contours forming the diagonals of the square, the upper and lower gratings being horizontal and the left and right being vertical, or (2) by an effort of will, as concentric squares, whereupon the phantom contours disappear. When the figure is viewed in the second way, only one or two squares are seen as complete squares, and this destroys the impression of gratings. If the subject has previously adapted to coloured gratings, he sees McCollough colours when he views the test pattern in the first way, but the colours disappear when he views it in the second.

Some recent work (Finke and Schmidt, 1977) claims that coloured after-effects can be produced when one part of the adapting stimulus, either the pattern or the colours, is not actually presented but is imagined by the subject. The subject then, when shown a test pattern consisting of orthogonal achromatic gratings, was required to make a forced choice discrimination in which he wrote down which grating seemed to him redder or greener. The authors compared the results to those obtained in the dichoptic experiment of MacKay and MacKay (1973), see chapter 5. With 'bar imagination', i.e. when alternate colours were presented but orthogonal gratings were imagined, a McCollough-like (negative) after-effect was recorded, comparable to the McCollough effect produced in the colour stimulated eye with dichoptic presentation. In other words, the imagined bars acted like bars presented to the non-colour stimulated eye in the dichoptic experiment. With 'colour imagination', i.e. when alternate orthogonal gratings were presented and the colours were imagined, a positive after-effect or reversed McCollough effect was recorded, comparable to the reversed McCollough effect produced dichoptically in the pattern stimulated eye: i.e. the imagined colours act like colours presented to the non-pattern stimulated eye in the dichoptic procedure.

I have to confess that when I repeated this experiment on myself the results were negative. Possibly the hypnotic effects of another person directing the proceedings are necessary to stimulate the imagination. What I might have done in a forced choice situation I cannot say, but certainly I saw no induced colours, even weak ones, of the strength that I am accustomed to measure. However, taking the experiment at its face value, and 144 subjects were tested by Finke and Schmidt, it is possible to make the following interpretation, as set out in the schema of table 18. When an external colour stimulus is coupled with *either* an external pattern stimulus or an internal pattern stimulus, which may be derived either from imagination or dichoptically through interocular transfer from an external pattern stimulus presented to the other eye, then a McCollough or *negative* after-effect is set up. This can be regarded as a forgetting mechanism designed to break an unwanted association between colour and pattern. If, on the other hand, an external pattern stimulus is coupled with an internal colour stimulus, which may be derived either from imagination or through interocular transfer from an external colour presented to

Table 18

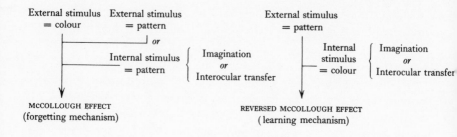

MCCOLLOUGH EFFECT
(forgetting mechanism)

REVERSED MCCOLLOUGH EFFECT
(learning mechanism)

the other eye, then a reversed McCollough or *positive* after-effect is set up. If the McCollough effect is a forgetting mechanism, then the reversed McCollough effect is a promoter of learning, tending to strengthen rather than weaken associations with pattern. Colour and pattern, then, are qualitatively different stimuli producing qualitatively different effects. It may not be merely a matter of convenience that written language, which requires to foster associations, is based on differences of pattern rather than of colour.

Purpose of the McCollough effect

Most workers who have studied the McCollough effect have tended to regard it as suitable material for laboratory experimentation rather than as a phenomenon with a definite function. It seems scarcely credible, however, that a visual effect which, in spite of its apparent weakness, results from the equivalent of a 50 per cent or greater suppression of a particular spectral wavelength and has the potentiality for enforcing this suppression stored in the brain for so long, should after all prove to be purely fortuitous with no *raison d'être*. Anstis (1975) has suggested that the role of the McCollough effect is to eliminate 'cross-talk, in the form of spuriously coloured edges etc.' in cortical units responding to more than one visual feature. This explanation, like many early ideas on the mechanism of the McCollough effect, leans rather heavily on the responses of individual colour-coded or direction-coded neurones. If a liability to 'cross-talk' or confusion between different types of visual stimulation really presents a problem to the brain, it is possible that more complex mechanisms including memory-like

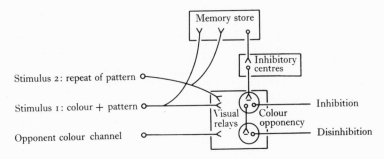

Fig. 45. McCollough effect. Hypothetical inhibitory basis.

processes could be made available to provide correction. Since, however, we do not know that the problem exists, and we do know that forgetting is an important function of the brain, the forgetting hypothesis seems to be for the moment more attractive. Because weak McCollough effects decay more slowly than strong ones the consequence will be to expunge more effectively from the record the minor and more trivial associations and to emphasise those of greater significance. (Slow decay = relatively high ME strengths = enhanced forgetting.) In this way, through selective forgetting a bias will be set up that will actually facilitate learning.

If this interpretation is correct, the evidence from the McCollough effect suggests that forgetting is achieved through inhibitory mechanisms, and learning through excitatory mechanisms involving acetylcholine. Little is known about how we normally come to forget irrelevant material, but there are good reasons for believing that cholinergic processes are involved in learning and memory (Alpern and Marriott, 1973; Vasko *et al.*, 1974). An anti-cholinergic drug such as hyoscine impairs the performance of a learned task in rats in a manner consistent with memory block (Deutsch, 1971). Anti-cholinergic drugs also produce memory impairment in man (Bignani and Rosić, 1971; Drachman and Leavitt, 1974). Choline acetyltransferase, the enzyme responsible for the synthesis of acetylcholine, and acetylcholinesterase are both said to be present in increased amounts in the temporal lobe cortex of animals with high learning ability (Ebel *et al.*, 1973; Mandel *et al.*, 1974). Stimulation of the reticular formation of the midbrain, which is the site of origin of ascending cholinergic pathways (Shute and Lewis, 1963, 1967), enhances memory storage in rats (Bloch *et al.*, 1970).

Lesions in the region of the ventral tegmental cholinergic pathway of Shute and Lewis, on the other hand, have been found to impair learning (Thompson and Hawkins, 1961; Olds and Hogberg, 1964; Santacana and Delacour, 1968). Electrocortical desynchronisation, which is produced by activation of the cholinergic system, may be necessary for memory consolidation (Thompson and Obrist, 1964; Koukkou and Lehmann, 1968). Total bilateral lesions of the globus pallidus produce loss of conditioned reflexes in cats which are then re-established, if at all, only with the greatest difficulty (Gambarian *et al.*, 1971). Such lesions, in addition to interfering with extra-pyramidal motor pathways, would destroy some of the cortico-petal cholinergic radiations and much of the cholinergic innervation of the lateral and ventral diencephalon.

At first sight it may seem paradoxical that the McCollough effect as a forgetting mechanism should involve a memory process – recognition at a subsequent presentation of the adapting pattern – to bring it into action. Less so, perhaps, if memory and forgetting are seen as opposite sides of the same coin, memory requiring increased cholinergic activity, and forgetting a swing of the balance away from cholinergic excitation and towards inhibition. A simple model of the McCollough effect as a process involving memory and inhibition is shown in fig. 45. At the first presentation of a pattern, the existence of an association with colour is recorded in the memory store. When the pattern is re-presented without the colour, the memory store having received the information activates an inhibitory mechanism which depresses the activity of neurones normally responsive to that colour at one or more visual relays. The opponent colour channel is disinhibited through another inhibitory link. If, in such a model, the 'memory store' is to be anything more than just a black box, it is necessary to probe deeper into what is known and what has been hypothesised about the nature of memory.

Holography and memory

It has been thought that a useful analogy for the processes by which memories are laid down and retrieved can be found in holography. Fig. 46 illustrates the principle of holography in a simple way. Light from a coherent source S, e.g. a laser, is reflected off an object OO′ (the path by which the light reaches the object is immaterial)

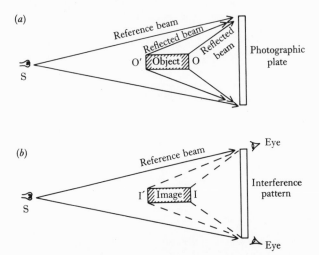

Fig. 46. Principle of holography. (*a*) Production of interference pattern with coherent light. The route by which the light reaches the object is unimportant. (*b*) Re-creation of object by reference beam. The light paths for the image to the eye are those which, in conjunction with the reference beam, will generate the interference pattern: i.e. they coincide with the original reflected beams from the object.

to reach a photographic plate of fine grain, where it interacts with light direct from the source to form an interference pattern. The light from the object is called the reflected beam, and the direct light from the coherent source the reference beam. The object is re-created as a virtual image II' when coherent, or nearly coherent light corresponding to the reference beam again falls on the photographic plate, and the observer looks through the interference pattern. Comparing the two diagrams it will be seen that in each case two elements of the system are required to create the third: in (1) the reference beam and the object create the interference pattern, and in (2) the reference beam and the interference pattern create the image. Different aspects of the object are recorded in different parts of the photographic plate, so that the image is seen in three dimensions. If two objects at different distances are contained in the hologram, they will exhibit true parallax as the observer moves his gaze across the plate. This can be compared with the false parallax that occurs in stereograms (chapter 4).

One of the attractions of holography as a paradigm for memory

(*a*)

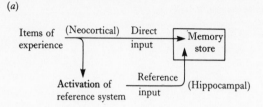

(*b*)

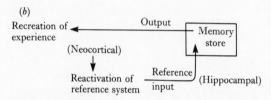

Fig. 47. Holography as a model for memory. (*a*) Formation of 'memory trace'. (*b*) Memory retrieval.

is the great economy of space that can be achieved through the recording of multiple holograms on a single plate. Two separate objects O_1 and O_2 will be represented on a hologram without overlap if at the photographic plate the angular distance θ between their centres is greater than the sum of their angular radii. If two exposures are made on a single plate, with O_2 occupying the same position as O_1 but the reference beam rotated through an angle θ for the second exposure, then if θ is greater than the sum of the angular radii of O_1 and O_2, separate non-overlapping images will be produced by the hologram when the reference beam is set to the same two positions.

To what extent, then, can holography be said to provide a valid analogy for memory? In one sense it must so do, because in each case an item of information is recorded in coded form (interference pattern, memory trace), which is stored and read out on a subsequent occasion. The important question is, is there in memory an analogue of the reference beam (fig. 47)? To begin to answer this, one must look at the connections of the part of the brain known to be essential to the laying down and retrieval of memories, namely the hippocampus.

The hippocampus and memory

The importance of the hippocampus in memory was first appreciated some thirty years ago when it was discovered that patients
treated for temporal lobe epilepsy by bilateral hippocampectomy
or, in cases where the hippocampus on the opposite side was
functionally damaged, by unilateral extirpation of the hippocampus, suffered a disability far greater than that with which they were
previously afflicted, namely an almost total and permanent inability
to lay down, or retrieve, new memories (Penfield and Milner, 1958;
Drachman and Ommaya, 1964). It can also be shown, though with
more difficulty, that hippocampal lesions produce an equivalent
of amnesia in animals (Iversen, 1976). The hippocampus receives
a cholinergic input (Shute and Lewis, 1963, 1966; Lewis and Shute,
1967; Lewis *et al.*, 1967) and projects extensively onto the
cholinergic midbrain reticular formation through the mammillo-
tegmental tract (Lewis and Shute, 1967). Through these
connections the hippocampus probably functions synergistically
with the cholinergic system (Lewis and Shute, 1967; Shute, 1973).
Hippocampal lesions depress cortical levels of acetylcholine (Pepeu
et al., 1973). Degeneration of the mammillary bodies, from which
the mammillo-tegmental tracts arise, is the classic lesion of Korsakoff amnesia associated with senility, alcoholism, etc. (Barbizet,
1963; Kahn and Crosby, 1972). Loss of conditioned reflexes in cats,
produced by globus pallidus lesions, also occur after hippocampal
damage (Gambarian *et al.*, 1972).

The hippocampus has the ability to concentrate heavy metals,
especially zinc; in the rat, the zinc content of the hippocampus is
three times that of the rest of the body (Fjerdingstad *et al.*, 1974*a*,
b). The zinc is located around the synaptic terminals of the
hippocampal input and may play a part in neural transmission.
Disulphiram ('antabuse') is a chelating agent and so sequesters
heavy metals, although it also affects catecholamine metabolism
and is believed to inhibit various enzymes including those responsible for oxidising alcohol. The effects of disulphiram on learning
are mainly depressive (Kleinrok *et al.*, 1970; Baru and Bozhko,
1970; Randt *et al.*, 1971; Osborn and Kerkut, 1972). The central
effects of zinc deficiency in man, e.g. anorexia, lethargy, emotional
lability, are not dissimilar from those resulting from alcoholism

(Henkin *et al.*, 1975). The hippocampal zinc may be replaced with lead in acute lead poisoning, especially in children.

The hippocampus may also be involved in autism (Hauser *et al.*, 1975). Children suffering from this condition may have an enlargement of one or both inferior horns of the lateral ventricle of the brain, as shown by pneumography, indicating an abnormality of the medial temporal lobe. There may be an abnormal temporal electroencephalogram. The hippocampus and amygdala are very sensitive to ischaemia and hypoxia, and there is often a history of birth injury. The symptoms include a failure of normal language development, an inability to relate to other people, an obsessive preoccupation with particular objects, and a sustained resistance to change in the environment. The last two can be compared with the 'perseveration' which is the most characteristic feature of hippocampal lesions in experimental animals. Hippocampecto-mised animals tend to persist with a particular line of behaviour even when it is not appropriate. Explanations that have been proposed for perseveration include the following (not all mutually exclusive): (*a*) impaired inhibition of stimulus–response bands (Douglas, 1967; Albert and Mah, 1973); (*b*) impaired habituation to novel stimuli (Kimble, 1968); (*c*) impaired familiarity dis-crimination (Gaffan, 1972, 1973); (*d*) hyper-reactivity to stimuli (Dalland, 1974); (*e*) enhanced experience of reward, enhanced incentive motivation (Brown *et al.*, 1969; Haddad and Rabe, 1969; Jackson and Gergen, 1970; Henke, 1975).

Vinogradova has proposed that the hippocampus acts as a comparator registering familiarity and novelty (Vinogradova, 1970; Vinogradova *et al.*, 1970). According to this hypothesis, the hippocampus receives two streams of information, one from the sensory system via the reticular formation and the other from the memory store via the entorhinal cortex. The two streams are compared within the hippocampus through the responses of two types of cells. One group, the 'I cells' or identity detectors are in a majority and are active when the two inputs match; when a mismatch occurs they became silent. The other group, 'A cells' or novelty detectors, are active when the inputs mismatch. They are responsible for the so-called 'orienting reaction' that occurs when an experimental animal finds itself in a new situation, supervening on the 'startle response'. As the stimulus becomes familiar the novelty detectors undergo habituation; meanwhile a memory trace is registered in the memory store as a result of information carried to the cingulate gyrus via the mammillo-thalamic tract, and reticular activity is damped down through the influence of the mammillo-tegmental projection.

The above account, which I hope represents adequately Vino-gradova's views, emphasises the fornix–mammillo-thalamic output from the hippocampus. It is far from certain, however, that this pathway is the most important one subserving memory in the ordinary sense (see Thompson and Hawkins, 1961) in spite of the role claimed for the mammillary bodies in Korsakoff's syndrome. More than half the fornix fibres terminate in the preoptic and hypothalamic regions and never reach the mammillary bodies, and it is possible that the projection to the cingulate gyrus is more concerned with emotive and visceral functions of the hippocampus. The major hippocampal output concerned with the laying down and retrieval of memories may be a direct one to the ipsilateral entorhinal cortex (the connections between entorhinal cortex and hippocampus are two-way: Votaw (1959, 1960); Hjorth-Simonsen (1971)) and a crossed pathway via the dorsal hippocampal com-missure to the entorhinal cortex of the opposite side. If there is an equivalent to the 'reference beam' of holography, it is perhaps to be seen in these hippocampo-entorhinal connections.

A model for the McCollough effect

The psychophysical experiments described in this work throw very little light on whereabouts in the visual system the McCollough effect is produced. Various features of the phenomenon, e.g. the retinal area specificity (Stromeyer, 1972b), the limited interocular transfer, the reversal of colours when the head is turned sideways, all seem to implicate the primary pathway between the retina and layer IV of the visual cortex, relaying in the lateral geniculate body. If, as has been argued, the basis of the after-effect is inhibition of colour-sensitive neurones, their inhibition could be produced at various levels and not necessary only at one. Similarly with eradication of the McCollough effect, in which, it has been suggested, cholinergic mechanisms may play an essential part. Acetylcholine is, predominantly at least, excitatory in the visual system, and is released when the midbrain reticular formation is

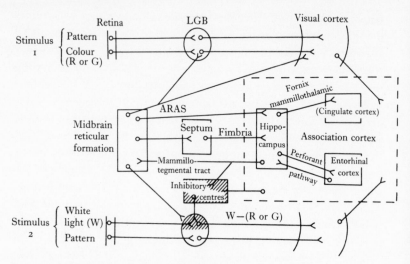

Fig. 48. Suggested model for McCollough effect: cf. fig. 45.

activated. Reticular stimulation depresses inhibition in the lateral geniculate body (Singer and Schmielau, 1976) and facilitates activity – and so, presumably, counters inhibition, in the visual cortex (Singer *et al.*, 1976). The onset of inhibition must be under the control of a memory link.

An attempt to show some of these interactions is made in fig. 48 – a more elaborate version of fig. 45 in which the 'memory store' box has been replaced by a reticulo-hippocampal–cortical system. Inhibition on a colour pathway is shown for convenience as occurring in the lateral geniculate body where many colour-coded cells are situated (Wiesel and Hubel, 1966), but this is not intended to exclude inhibition elsewhere. Complex as the schema is, it is still an over-simplification, since no attempt has been made to illustrate, for instance, the opposed cholinergic and dopaminergic inputs to the hippocampus, the presence of intrinsic gabaminergic inhibitory interneurones within the hippocampus, etc. The model still contains a 'black box' representing the source of the inhibition. The drug experiments so far performed simply show that any procedure which raises the level of central inhibition tends to enhance the McCollough effect. There is so far no indication as to which inhibitory neurotransmitter or neurotransmitters are responsible for producing the McCollough effect and resisting its decay, nor where the neurones releasing them are located. The elucidation of these, and indeed many other points requires further work. There would seem to be no inseparable difficulty in setting up a McCollough effect in an experimental animal with good colour vision such as a monkey and in looking for changes in the activity of colour-coded cells. Perhaps this is the direction for further advance.

REFERENCES

Albert, D. J. and Mah, C. J. (1973) Passive avoidance deficit with septal lesions: disturbance of response inhibition or response acquisition? *Physiol. Behav.* **11**, 205–13.

Alpern, H. P. and Marriott, D. J. (1973) Short-term memory: facilitation and disruption with cholinergic agents. *Physiol. Behav.* **11**, 571–5.

Amure, B. O. (1978) Nicotine and the decay of the McCollough effect. *Vision Res.* **18**, 1449–51.

Anstis, S. M. (1975) What does visual perception tell us about visual coding? In *Handbook of Psychobiology* (M. S. Gazzaniga and C. Blakemore, eds.) chapter 9. New York: Academic Press.

Armitage, A. K., Hall, G. H. and Morrison, C. F. (1968) Pharmacological basis for the tobacco smoking habit. *Nature, Lond.* **217**, 331–4.

Barbizet, J. (1963) Defect of memorizing of hippocampal–mammillary origin. *J. Neurol. Neurosurg. Psychiat.* **26**, 127–35.

Baru, A. M. and Bozhko, G. Kh. (1970) Effect of some inhibitors and metabolites of catecholamine metabolism on the fixation and reproduction of memory traces. *Bull. exp. Biol. Med.* **70**, 1017–20.

Bhagat, B. (1970) Influence of chronic administration of nicotine on the turnover and metabolism of noradrenaline in the rat brain. *Psychopharmacologia* **18**, 325–32.

Biel, J. H. (1970) Structure–activity relationships of amphetamine and derivatives. In *Amphetamines and Related Compounds* (E. Costa and S. Garattini, eds.). New York: Raven Press.

Bignani, G. and Rosić, N. (1971) The nature of disinhibiting phenomena caused by central cholinergic muscarinic blockade. In *Advances in Neuropsychopharmacology* (O. Vinar, Z. Votava and P. B. Bradley, eds.). Amsterdam: North-Holland.

Blakemore, C. and van Sluyters, R. (1974) Reversal of the physiological effects of monocular deprivation in kittens: further evidence for a sensitive period. *J. Physiol., Lond.* **237**, 195–216.

Bloch, V., Deweer, B. and Hennevin, E. (1970) Suppression de l'amnésie retrograde et consolidation d'un apprentissage à essai unique par stimulation réticulaire. *Physiol. Behav.* **5**, 1215–41.

Bohus, B., Gispen, W.-H. and de Wied, D. (1973) Effect of lysine vasopressin and ACTH on conditioned avoidance behaviour of hypophysectomized rats. *Neuroendocrinology* **11**, 137–43.

Bowman, R. (1966) Magnesium pemoline and behavior. *Science, N.Y.* **153**, 902.

Bradbury, M. W. B., Burden, J., Dicker, A., Hillhouse, E., Jones, M. T. and Philbrick, D. (1973) Stimulation of rat hypothalamus *in vitro. J. Physiol., Lond.* **234**, 74P.

Breitmeyer, B. G. and Cooper, L. A. (1972) Frequency-specific colour adaptation in the human visual system. *Percept. & Psychophys.* **11**, 95–6.

Brown, T. S., Kaufmann, P. G. and Marco, L. A. (1969) The hippocampus and response perseveration in the cat. *Brain Res.* **12**, 86–98.

Bryant, H. C. and Jarmie, N. (1974) The glory. *Scientific American* **231**, 60–71.

Burns, J. T., House, R. F., Feusch, F. C. and Miller, J. G. (1967) Effects of magnesium pemoline and dextroamphetamine on human learning. *Science, N.Y.* **155**, 849–51.

Campbell, F. W., Hess, R. F. and Shute, C. C. D. (1978a) The McCollough effect and amblyopia. *J. Physiol., Lond., Proceedings* (in press).

Campbell, F. W., Hess, R. F., Watson, P. G. and Banks, R. (1978b) Preliminary results of a physiologically based treatment of amblyopia. *Brit. J. Ophthal.* (in press).

Campbell, F. W., Shute, C. C. D. and Tapp, R. L. (1975) Rapid measurement of mean corpuscular diameter. *J. Physiol., Lond.* **247**, 6P.

Corcoran, D. W. J. and Houston, T. G. (1977) Is the lemon test an index of arousal level? *Br. J. Psychol.* **68**, 361–4.

Crossland, J. (1971) Neurohumeral substances and drug abstinence syndrome. In *Advances in Neuropsychopharmacology* (O. Vinar, Z. Votava and P. B. Bradley, eds.). Amsterdam: North-Holland.

Crow, J. J. (1972) A map of the rat mesencephalon for electrical self stimulation. *Brain Res.* **3**, 265–73.

Dahlström, A. and Fuxe, K. (1964) Evidence for the existence of monoamine-containing neurones in the central nervous system. *Acta physiol. scand.* **62**, suppl. 232.

Dalland, T. (1974) Stimulus perseveration of rats with septal lesions. *Physiol. Behav.* **12**, 1957–61.

Darragh, P. J., Gaskin, A. J. and Sanders, J. V. (1976) Opals. *Scientific American* **234**, April, 84–95.

Deutsch, J. A. (1971) The cholinergic synapse and the site of memory. *Science, N.Y.* **174**, 778–94.

De Valois, R. L., Abramov, I. and Jacobs, G. H. (1966) Analysis of response patterns of LGN cells. *J. opt. Soc. Am.* **56**, 966–77.

Douglas, R. J. (1967) The hippocampus and behaviour. *Psychol. Bull.* **67**, 416–42.

Drachman, D. A. and Leavitt, J. (1974) Human memory and the cholinergic system: relationship to aging? *Arch. Neurol.* **30**, 113–21.

Drachman, D. A. and Ommaya, A. K. (1964) Memory and the hippocampal complex. *Arch. Neurol.* **10**, 411–25.

Drew, W. G. and Miller, L. L. (1974) Cannabis: neural mechanisms and behaviour – a theoretical review. *Pharmacology* **11**, 12–32.

Duffy, F. H., Snodgrass, S. R., Burchifiel, J. L. and Conway, J. L. (1976) Bicuculline reversal of deprivation amblyopia in the cat. *Nature, Lond.* **260**, 256–7.

Ebel, A., Hermetet, J. C. and Mandel, P. (1973) Comparative study of acetylcholinesterase and choline acetyltransferase enzyme activity in brain of DBA and C57 mice. *Nature (New Biol.) Lond.* **242**, 56–8.

Favreau, O. E. and Cornwallis, M. C. (1976) Negative after effects in visual perception. *Scientific American* **235**, December, 42–8.

Feinberg, G. (1968) Light. *Scientific American* **219**, September, 50–9.

Finke, R. A. and Schmidt, M. J. (1977) Orientation-specific colour after-effects following imagination. *J. exp. Psychol. Human Perc. & Perf.* **3**, 599–606.

Fjerdingstad, E., Danscher, G. and Fjerdingstad, E. J. (1974*a*) Zinc content in hippocampus and whole brain of normal rats. *Brain Res.* **79**, 338–42.

Fjerdingstad, E. J., Danscher, G. and Fjerdingstad, E. (1974*b*) Hippocampus: selective concentration of lead in the normal rat brain. *Brain Res.* **80**, 350–4.

Francis, M. G. and Peaslee, M. H. (1974) Effects of social stress on pituitary melanocyte stimulating hormone activity in male mice. *Neuroendocrinology* **16**, 1–7.

Fulder, S. (1976) *About Ginseng*. Wellingborough: Thorsons.

Fulder, S. (1977) Ginseng: useless root or subtle medicine? *New Scientist* **73**, 138–9.

Fuxe, K. (1965) The distribution of monoamine terminals in the central nervous system. *Acta physiol. scand.* **64**, suppl. 247, 37.

Gaffan, D. (1972) Loss of recognition memory in rats with lesions of the fornix. *Neuropsychologia* **10**, 327–41.

Gaffan, D. (1973) Inhibitory gradients and behavioural contrast in rats with lesions of the fornix. *Physiol. Behav.* **11**, 215–20.

Gähwiler, B. H. (1976) Diazepam and chlordiazepoxide: powerful GABA antagonists in explants of rat cerebellum. *Brain Res.* **197**, 176–9.

Gambarian, L. S., Garibian, A. A., Sarkisian, J. S. and Ganodian, V. O. (1971) Conditional motor reflexes in cats with damage to the globus pallidus. *Exp. Brain Res.* **12**, 92–104.

Gambarian, L. S., Koval, I. N., Garibian, A. A. and Sarkisian, J. S. (1972) Conditional motor reflexes in cats with damage to the hippocampus. *Exp. Brain Res.* **15**, 15–28.

Gerlach, J. L. and McEwen, B. S. (1972) Rat brain binds adrenal steroid hormone: radioautography of hippocampus with corticosterone. *Science, N.Y.* **175**, 1133–6.

Glasky, A. J. and Simon, L. N. (1966) Magnesium pemoline: enhancement of brain RNA polymerases. *Science, N.Y.* **151**, 702–3.

Gray, J. A. (1964) *Pavlov's Typology*. Oxford: Pergamon.

Greengard, P., McAfee, D. A. and Kebabian, J. W. (1972) On the mechanism of action of cyclic AMP and its role in synaptic transmission. *Advances in Cyclic Nucleotide Res.* **1**, 337–55.

Haddad, R. K. and Rabe, A. (1969) Modified temporal behaviour in rats after large hippocampal lesions. *Exp. Neurol.* **23**, 310–17.

Hall, G. H. and Turner, D. M. (1972) Effects of nicotine on the release of ³H-noradrenaline from the hypothalamus. *Biochem. Pharmacol.* **21**, 1829–38.

Hauser, S. L., DeLong, G. R. and Rosman, N. P. (1975) Pneumographic findings in the infantile autism syndrome: a correlation with temporal lobe disease. *Brain* **98**, 667–88.

Hay, J. C., Pick, H. L. and Rosser, E. (1963) Adaptation to chromatic aberration by the human visual system. *Science, N.Y.* **141**, 167–9.

Henke, P. G. (1975) Septal lesions and the extinction of incentive-motivation. *Physiol. Behav.* **15**, 537–42.

Henkin, R. I., Patten, B. M., Re, P. K. and Bronzert, D. A. (1975) A syndrome of acute zinc loss. Cerebellar dysfunction, mental changes, anorexia, and taste and smell dysfunction. *Arch. Neurol.* **32**, 745–51.

Hillhouse, E. W., Burden, J. and Jones, M. T. (1975) The effect of various putative neurotransmitters on the release of corticotrophin releasing hormone from the hypothalamus of the rat *in vitro*. *Neuroendocrinology* **17**, 1–11.

Hjorth-Simonsen, A. (1971) Hippocampal efferents to the ipsilateral entorhinal area: an experimental study in the rat. *J. comp. Neurol.* **142**, 417–38.

Holding, D. H. and Jones, P. D. (1976) Delayed one-trial extinction of the McCollough effect. *Quart. J. exp. Psychol.* **28**, 683–7.

Hubel, D. H. and Wiesel, T. N. (1959) Receptive fields of single neurons in the cat's striate cortex. *J. Physiol., Lond.* **148**, 574–91.

Hubel, D. H. and Wiesel, T. N. (1962) Receptive fields, binocular interaction, and functional architecture in the cat's visual cortex. *J. Physiol., Lond.* **160**, 106–23.

Hubel, D. H. and Wiesel, T. N. (1968) Receptive fields and functional architecture of the monkey striate cortex. *J. Physiol., Lond.* **195**, 215–43.

Hubel, D. H. and Wiesel, T. N. (1970) The period of susceptibility to the physiological effects of unilateral eye closure in kittens. *J. Physiol., Lond.* **206**, 419–36.

Iversen, S. (1976) Do hippocampal lesions produce amnesia in animals? *Int. Rev. Neurobiol.* **19**, 1–49.

Jackson, F. B. and Gergen, J. A. (1970) Acquisition of operant schedules by squirrel monkeys lesioned in the hippocampal area. *Physiol. Behav.* **5**, 543–7.

Jenkins, B. and Ross J. (1977) McCollough effect depends on perceived organization. *Perception* **6**, 399–400.

Jones, P. D. and Holding, D. H. (1975) Extremely long-term persistence of the McCollough effect. *J. exp. Psychol. Human Perc. & Perf.* **1**, 323–7.

Julesz, B. (1971) *Foundations of Cyclopean Perception.* Chicago: University of Chicago Press.

Kahn, E. A. and Crosby, E. C. (1972) Korsakoff's syndrome associated with surgical lesions involving the mammillary bodies. *Neurology* 22, 117–25.

Kanai, T. and Szerb, J. C. (1965) Mesencephalic reticular activating system and cortical acetylcholine output. *Nature, Lond.* 205, 80–2.

Kasamatsu, T. and Pettigrew, J. D. (1976) Depletion of brain catecholamines: failure of ocular dominance shift after monocular occlusion in kittens. *Science, N.Y.* 194, 206–9.

Kimble, D. P. (1968) Hippocampus and internal inhibition. *Psychol. Bull.* 70, 285–95.

Kleinrok, Z., Zebrowska, I. and Weilosz, M. (1970) Some central effects of diethyldithiocarbonate administered intraventricularly in rats. *Neuropharmacology* 9, 451–5.

Knights, R. M. and Viets, C. A. (1975) Effects of pemoline on hyperactive boys. *Pharm. Biochem. Behav.* 3, 1107–14.

Kohler, I. (1962) Experiments with goggles. *Scientific American* 206, May, 62–72.

Koukkou, M. and Lehmann, D. (1968) EEG and memory storage in sleep experiments with humans. *Electroenceph. clin. Neurophysiol.* 25, 455–62.

Kozhechkin, S. N. and Ostrovskaya, R. V. (1977) Are benzodiazepines GABA antagonists? *Nature, Lond.* 269, 72–3.

Kratz, K. E., Spear, P. D. and Smith, D. C. (1976) Postcritical-period reversal of effects of monocular deprivation on striate cortex cells in the rat. *J. Neurophysiol.* 39, 501–11.

Krnjević, K. and Phillis, J. W. (1963a) Acetylcholine-sensitive cells in the cerebral cortex. *J. Physiol., Lond.* 166, 296–327.

Krnjević, K. and Phillis, J. W. (1963b) Pharmacological properties of acetylcholine-sensitive cells in the cerebral cortex. *J. Physiol., Lond.* 166, 328–50.

Krnjević, K. and Phillis, J. W. (1963c) Actions of certain amines on cerebral cortical neurones. *Brit. J. Pharmacol.* 20, 471–90.

Land, E. H. (1977) The retinex theory of colour vision. *Scientific American* 237, December, 108–29.

Land, M. F. (1966) A multilayer interference reflector in the eye of the scallop, *Pecten maximus*. *J. exp. Biol.* 45, 433–47.

Leppman, P. K. (1973) Spatial frequency dependent chromatic after-effects. *Nature, Lond.* 242, 411–12.

Lewis, P. R. and Shute, C. C. D. (1967) The cholinergic limbic system: projections to the hippocampal formation, medial cortex, nuclei of the ascending cholinergic reticular system, and subfornical organ and supra-optic crest. *Brain* 90, 521–40.

Lewis, P. R. and Shute, C. C. D. (1978) Cholinergic pathways in CNS. Chapter 6 in *Handbook of Psychopharmacology* vol. 9 (L. L. Iversen, S. D. Iversen and S. H. Snyder, eds.). New York: Plenum.

Lewis, P. R., Shute, C. C. D. and Silver, A. (1967) Confirmation from choline acetylase analyses of a massive cholinergic innervation to the rat hippocampus. *J. Physiol., Lond.* 191, 215–24.

Lippa, A. S., Antelman, S. M., Fisher, A. E. and Canfield, D. R. (1973) Neurochemical mediation of reward: a significant role for dopamine? *Pharmac. Biochem. Behav.* **1**, 23–8.

Lovegrove, W. J. and Over, R. (1972) Colour adaptation of spatial frequency detectors in the human visual system. *Science, N.Y.* **176**, 541–3.

McCarter, A. and Silver, A. I. (1977) The McCollough effect: a classical conditioning phenomenon? *Vision Res.* **17**, 317–19.

McCollough, C. (1965) Color adaptation of edge-detectors in the human visual system. *Science, N.Y.* **149**, 1115–16.

MacKay, D. M. and MacKay, V. (1973) Orientation-sensitive after-effects of dichoptically presented colour and form. *Nature, Lond.* **242**, 477–9.

MacKay, D. M. and MacKay, V. (1974) The time course of the McCollough effect and its physiological implications. *J. Physiol., Lond.* **237**, 38–9P.

MacKay, D. M. and MacKay, V. (1975a) Dichoptic induction of McCollough-type effects. *Quart. J. exp. Psychol.* **27**, 225–33.

MacKay, D. M. and MacKay, V. (1975b) What causes decay of pattern-contingent chromatic after-effects? *Vision Res.* **15**, 462–4.

MacKay, V. and MacKay, D. M. (1977) Multiple orientation-contingent chromatic after-effects. *Quart. J. exp. Psychol.* **29**, 203–18.

Mandel, P., Ayad, G., Hermetet, J. C. and Ebel, A. (1974) Correlation between choline acetyltransferase activity and learning ability in different mice strains and their offspring. *Brain Res.* **72**, 65–70.

Marx, J. L. (1975) Learning and behaviour. II. The hypothalamic peptides. *Science, N.Y.* **190**, 544–5.

Masland, R. H. and Ames, A. (1976) Responses to acetylcholine of ganglion cells in an isolated mammalian retina. *J. Neurophysiol.* **39**, 1220–35.

Masland, R. H. and Livingstone, C. J. (1976) Effect of stimulation with light on synthesis and release of acetylcholine by an isolated mammalian retina. *J. Neurophysiol.* **39**, 1210–19.

Matthews, E. K. and Quilliam, J. P. (1964) Effects of central depressant drugs on acetylcholine release. *Br. J. Pharmac.* **22**, 415–40.

Mayhew, J. E. W. and Anstis, S. M. (1972) Movement after-effects contingent on colour, intensity and pattern. *Percept. & Psychophys.* **12**, 77–85.

Mikaelian, H. H. (1974) Interocular generalization of orientation specific color after-effects. *Vision Res.* **15**, 661–3.

Moriarty, G. C., Halmi, N. S. and Moriarty, C. M. (1975) The effect of stress on the cytology and immunocytochemistry of pars intermedia cells in the rat pituitary. *Endocrinology* **96**, 1426–36.

Murch, G. M. (1969) Size judgments of McCollough afterimages. *J. exp. Psychol.* **81**, 44–8.

Murch, G. M. (1972) Binocular relationships in a size and colour orientation specific after-effect. *J. exp Psychol.* **93**, 30–4.

Murch, G. M. (1976) Classical conditioning of the McCollough effect: temporal parameters. *Vision Res.* **16**, 615–19.

Murch, G. M. (1977) A reply to McCarter and Silver. *Vision Res.* **17**, 321–2.

Murch, G. M. and Hirsch, J. (1972) The McCollough effect created by complementary afterimages. *Am. J. Psychol.* **85**, 241–7.

Muset, P. P., Ramia, J. and Martin-Esteve, J. (1967) Action of pemoline on RNA metabolism in the brain. *Nature, Lond.* **215**, 522–3.

Newton, I. (1730) *Opticks*, 4th ed., reprinted 1952. New York: Dover Publications.

Noell, W. K. and Lasansky, A. (1959) Effects of electrophoretically applied drugs and electrical currents on the ganglian cells of the retina. *Fed. Proc. Fed. Am. Soc. exp. Biol.* **18**, 115.

Olds, M. E. and Hogberg, D. (1964) Subcortical lesions and maze retention in the rat. *Exp. Neurol.* **10**, 296–304.

Osborn, R. H. and Kerkut, G. A. (1977) Inhibition of noradrenaline biosynthesis and its effects on learning in rats. *Comp. gen. Pharmac.* **3**, 359–62.

Padgham, C. A. (1965) After images as a means of investigating rods and cones. In *Colour Vision* (A. V. S. de Reuck and J. Knight, eds.). London: Churchill.

Paton, W. D. M., Vizi, E. S. and Aboo Zar, M. (1971) The mechanism of acetylcholine release from parasympathetic nerves. *J. Physiol., Lond.* **215**, 819–48.

Pedler, C. (1963) The fine structure of the tapetum cellulosum. *Exp. Eye Res.* **2**, 189–95.

Penfield, W. and Milner, B. (1958) Memory deficit produced by bilateral lesions in the hippocampal zone. *Arch. Neurol. Psychiat.* **79**, 475–97.

Pepeu, G., Mulas, A. and Mulas, M. L. (1973) Changes in the acetylcholine content in the rat brain after lesions of the septum, fimbria and hippocampus. *Brain Res.* **57**, 153–64.

Pettigrew, J. D. and Kasamatsu, T. (1978) Local perfusion of noradrenaline maintains visual cortical plasticity. *Nature, Lond.* **271**, 761–3.

Phillips, A. G. and Fibiger, M. C. (1973) Dopaminergic and noradrenergic substrates of positive reinforcement: differential effects of *d*- and *l*-amphetamine. *Science, N.Y.* **179**, 575–7.

Piggins, D. J. and Leppman, P. K. (1973) Role of retinal image motion in evoking the McCollough effect. *Nature (New Biol.) Lond.,* **245**, 255–6.

Plotnikoff, N. (1966) Magnesium pemoline: enhancement of learning and memory of a conditioned avoidance response. *Science, N.Y.* **151**, 703–4.

Poincaré, H. (1905) Science and Hypothesis (trans. W. J. G.) chapter 6. London: Walter Scott Publishing Co.

Ramachandran, V. S. (1976) Learning-like phenomena in stereopsis. *Nature, Lond.* **262**, 382–4.

Randt, C. T., Quartermain, D., Goldstein, M. and Anagnoste, B. (1971) Norephinephrine biosynthesis inhibition: effects on memory in mice. *Science, N.Y.* **172**, 498–9.

Rhees, R. W., Grosser, B. I. and Stevens, W. (1975) Effect of steroid competition and time on the uptake of ^{3}H-corticosterone in the rat brain: an autoradiographic study. *Brain Res.* **83**, 293–300.

Riggs, L. A. (1973) Curvature as a feature of pattern vision. *Science, N.Y.* **181**, 1070–2.

Riggs, L. A., White, K. D. and Eimas, P. D. (1974) Establishment and decay of orientation-contingent after effects of colour. *Percept. & Psychophys.* **16**, 535–42.

Robison, G. A., Butcher, R. W. and Sutherland, E. W. (1971) *Cyclic AMP.* New York: Academic Press.

Rozhdestvenskaya, V. I. (1955) An attempt to determine the strength of the process of excitation through features of its irradiation and concentration in the visual analyser. In *Pavlov's Typology* (J. A. Gray, ed.). Oxford: Pergamon.

Sandman, C. A., Kastin, A. J. and Schally, A. V. (1973) Neuroendocrine responses to physical and psychological stress. *J. comp. Physiol. Psychol.* **84**, 386–90.

Santacana, M. P. and Delacour, J. (1968) Effets, chez le rat, des lesions de la zona incerta et des corps mamillaires, sur un conditionnement defensif. *Neuropsychologia* **6**, 115–24.

Satinsky, D. (1967) Pharmacological responsiveness of lateral geniculate nucleus neurones. *Int. J. Neuropharmacol.* **6**, 387–97.

Shute, C. C. D. (1973) Cholinergic pathways of the brain. In *Surgical Approaches in Psychiatry* (L. V. Laitinen and K. E. Livingston, eds.), pp. 282–92. Lancaster: MTP.

Shute, C. C. D. (1974) Haidinger's brushes and predominant orientation of collagen in corneal stroma. *Nature, Lond.* **250**, 163–4.

Shute, C. C. D. (1975) Chemical transmitter systems in the brain. In *Modern Trends in Neurology* (D. Williams, ed.) pp. 183–203. London: Butterworths.

Shute, C. C. D. (1976) The 'blue moon' phenomenon. *Weather* **31**, 292–6.

Shute, C. C. D. (1977a) The formation of a 'glory'. *Weather* **32**, 64–6.

Shute, C. C. D. (1977b) A device for measuring the McCollough effect (ME) using polarised light. *J. Physiol., Lond.* **265**, 2–3P.

Shute, C. C. D. (1977c) Strength and decay of McCollough effects. *J. Physiol., Lond.* **268**, 34–5P.

Shute, C. C. D. (1977d) Interocular influences revealed by the McCollough effect. *J. Physiol., Lond.* **269**, 28–9P.

Shute, C. C. D. (1978) Influence of centrally active drugs on the McCollough effect (ME). *J. Physiol., Lond.* **278**, 47P.

Shute, C. C. D. and Lewis, P. R. (1961) The use of cholinesterase techniques combined with operative procedures to follow nervous pathways in the brain. *Biblphia anat.* **2**, 34–49.

Shute, C. C. D. and Lewis, P. R. (1963) Cholinesterase-containing systems of the brain of the rat. *Nature, Lond.* **199**, 1160–4.

Shute, C. C. D. and Lewis, P. R. (1966) Electron microscopy of cholinergic terminals and acetylcholinesterase-containing neurones in the hippocampal formation of the rat. *Z. Zellforsch.* **69**, 334–43.

Shute, C. C. D. and Lewis, P. R. (1967) The ascending cholinergic reticular system: neocortical, olfactory and subcortical projections. *Brain* **90**, 447–520.

Sigel, C. and Nachmias, J. (1975) A re-evaluation of curvature-specific chromatic after-effects. *Vision Res.* **15**, 829–36.

Singer, W. and Schmielau, F. (1976) The effect of reticular stimulation on binocular inhibition in the cat lateral geniculate body. *Exp. Brain Res.* **25**, 221–3.

Singer, W., Tretter, F. and Cynader, M. (1976) The effect of reticular stimulation on spontaneous and evoked activity in the cat visual cortex. *Brain Res.* **102**, 71–90.

Skowbo, D., Gentry, T., Timney, B. and Morant, R. B. (1974) The McCollough effect: influence of several kinds of visual stimulation on decay rate. *Percept. & Psychophys.* **16**, 47–9.

Skowbo, D., Timney, B. N., Gentry, T. A. and Morant, R. B. (1975) McCollough effects: experimental findings and theoretical accounts. *Psychol. Bull.* **82**, 497–510.

Spehlmann, R. (1963) Acetylcholine and prostigmine electrophoresis at visual cortex neurones. *J. Neurophysiol.* **26**, 127–39.

Spehlmann, R. (1971) Acetylcholine and the synaptic transmission of non-specific impulses to the visual cortex. *Brain* **94**, 139–50.

Spehlmann, R. and Downes, K. (1974) The effects of acetylcholine and of synaptic stimulation on the sensorimotor cortex of cats. I. Neuronal responses to stimulation of the reticular formation. *Brain Res.* **74**, 229–42.

Spehlmann, R. and Smathers, C. C. (1974) The effects of acetylcholine and of synaptic stimulation on the sensorimotor cortex of cats. II. Comparison of the neuronal responses to reticular and other stimuli. *Brain Res.* **74**, 243–53.

Steiner, F. A. and Felix, D. (1976) Antagonistic effects of GABA and benzodiazepines on vestibular and cerebellar neurones. *Nature, Lond.* **260**, 346–7.

Straschill, M. (1968) Actions of drugs on single neurones in the cat's retina. *Vision Res.* **8**, 35–47.

Stratton, L. O. and Kastin, A. J. (1973) Melanocyte stimulating hormone in learning and extinction of two problems. *Physiol. Behav.* **10**, 689–92.

Stromeyer, C. F. (1969) Further studies of the McCollough effect. *Percept. & Psychophys.* **6**, 105–10.

Stromeyer, C. F. (1971) McCollough effect analogues of two-color projections. *Vision Res.* **11**, 969–78.

Stromeyer, C. F. (1972a) Contour-contingent colour after-effects: spatial frequency specificity. *Vision Res.* **12**, 717–32.

Stromeyer, C. F. (1972b) Contour-contingent colour after-effects: retinal area specificity. *Am. J. Psychol.* **85**, 227–35.

Stromeyer, C. F. (1974) Curvature detectors in human vision? *Science, N.Y.* **184**, 1199–200.

Stromeyer, C. F. and Mansfield, R. (1970) Coloured after-effects produced with moving edges. *Percept. Psychophys.* **7**, 108–14.

Suria, A. and Costa, E. (1975) Action of diazepam, dibutyryl cGMP and GABA on presynaptic nerve terminals in bullfrog sympathetic ganglia. *Brain Res.* **87**, 102–6.

Teft, L. W. and Clark, F. T. (1968) The effects of stimulus density on orientation specific after-effects of color adaptation. *Psychonomic Sci.* **11**, 265–6.

Thompson, L. W. and Obrist, W. D. (1964) EEG correlates of verbal learning and overlearning. *Electroenceph. clin. Neurophysiol.* **16**, 332–42.

Thompson, R. and Hawkins, W. F. (1961) Memory uneffected by mamillary body lesions in the rat. *Exp. Neurol.* **3**, 189–96.

Torda, C. and Wolff, H. G. (1952) Effect of pituitary hormones, cortisone and adrenalectomy on some aspects of neuromuscular function and acetylcholine synthesis. *Am. J. Physiol.* **169**, 140–9.

Trabucci, M., Cheney, D., Racagni, G. and Costa, E. (1974) Involvement of brain cholinergic mechanisms in the action of chlorpromazine. *Nature, Lond.* **249**, 664–6.

Uhlarik, J. J. and Osgood, A. G. (1974) The role of some spatial parameters of gratings on the McCollough effect. *Percept. & Psychophys.* **15**, 524–8.

Vasko, M. R., Domino, L. E. and Domino, E. F. (1974) Differential effects of D-amphetamine on brain acetylcholine in young, adult and geriatric rats. *Eur. J. Pharmacol.* **27**, 145–7.

Versteeg, D. H. G. (1973) Effect of two ACTH-analogs on noradrenaline metabolism in rat brain. *Brain Res.* **49**, 483–5.

Vinogradova, O. S. (1970) Registration of information and the limbic system. In *Short-term Changes in Neural Activity and Behaviour* (G. Horn and R. A. Hinde, eds.). Cambridge University Press.

Vinogradova, O. S., Semyonova, T. P. and Konovalov, V. Ph. (1970) Trace phenomena in single neurones of hippocampus and mammillary bodies. In *Biology of Memory* (K. H. Pribram and D. E. Broadbent, eds.). New York: Academic Press.

Votaw, C. L. (1959) Certain functional and anatomical relations of the cornu ammonis of the macaque monkey. I. Functional relations. *J. comp. Neurol.* **112**, 353–82.

Votaw, C. L. (1960) Certain functional and anatomical relations of the cornu ammonis of the macaque monkey. II. Anatomical relations. *J. comp. Neurol.* **114**, 283–93.

Wallach, M. B. and Gershon, S. (1972) The induction of antagonism of central nervous system stimulant-induced stereotyped behaviour in the cat. *Eur. J. Pharmacol.* **18**, 22–6.

White, K. D. (1976) Luminance as a parameter in establishment and testing of the McCollough effect. *Vision Res.* **15**, 297–302.

White, K. D. (1977) Summation of successively established orientation-contingent colour after-effects. *Percept. & Psychophys.* **22**, 123–36.

Wiesel, T. N. and Hubel, D. H. (1966) Spatial and chromatic interactions in the lateral geniculate body of the rhesus monkey. *J. Neurophysiol.* **29**, 1115–56.

Young, T. (1802) Account of some cases of the production of colours. *Phil. Trans. Roy. Soc.* pp. 387–97.

AUTHOR INDEX

SUBJECT INDEX

Bold figures indicate figures or tables